"An indispensable handbook"

"This is a must read for anyone concerned about diabetes. It is an indispensable handbook that provides a wealth of information on diet, dietary supplements, and methods you can use to help treat your diabetes. This book is the key to a comprehensive treatment program that even your doctor may not know about!"

Marcia Zimmerman, MEd, CN
Bestselling Author of *7-Color Cuisine*

"Provides sound, practical advice"

"In his book, health researcher and educator Gene Bruno provides a completely up-to-date, thorough, and extensively researched approach to dealing with this epidemic disease. In his characteristic manner, Gene lays out his material in an easy-to-understand manner, and provides sound, practical advice for managing blood sugar disorders. I have come to expect the highest scholarship from Gene Bruno, and that is exactly what he delivers here. This is a highly valuable h

Chris Kil
Bestselling Author of

D1565332

"Timely and comprehensive"

"Gene Bruno's book is timely and comprehensive. A valuable resource for anyone with diabetes, this book also outlines a forward-thinking approach to using dietary supplements and complementary therapies that may well enlighten healthcare providers. Its scientific grounding and layman's language will help individuals take control of their total diabetic healthcare plan—in conversation with health professionals. "

Johanna Arnone
Publisher of *Taste for Life Magazine*

"Highly recommend"

"This book offers both the lay and professional reader a comprehensive, medically grounded approach for the holistic treatment of one of the world's modern health plagues: Diabetes. It provides a step-by-step road map for understanding and managing Diabetes as simply an imbalance of diet, nutrition and exercise rather than a life long curse with no foreseeable resolution. Gene offers hope and advice that very few physicians can even offer, in a concise, well organized and readable format. I highly recommend this book as a manual for patients already diagnosed with diabetes."

Keith R. DeOrio, M.D.
Bestselling Author of *The New Millennium Diet Revolution*

"A great self-help guide"

"Gene has put together a great self-help guide to blood sugar regulation and metabolic syndrome that provides a great and easy to grasp review of the various diets, herbs, and nutritional supplements that are of benefit for sugar control. Considering the incredibly negative impact that spiking blood sugar and insulin levels have on human physiology, this text should be a welcomed addition to the natural health care literature."

Roy Upton, Registered Herbalist
President of the American Herbal Pharmacopoeia

"Evidence-based information"

"In this book, Gene Bruno has demonstrated his ability to gather evidence-based information and present it in an organized manner. I continue to rely on Mr. Bruno for issues regarding my own health care and that of my patients."

Dr. Arthur M. Presser
President of Huntington College of Health Sciences
Author of *Pharmacists Guide to Medicinal Herbs*

A GUIDE TO
COMPLEMENTARY
TREATMENTS FOR
DIABETES

GENE BRUNO, MS, MHS

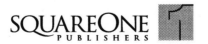

SQUAREONE
PUBLISHERS

The information and advice contained in this book are based
upon the research and the personal and professional experiences of
the author. They are not intended as a substitute for consulting with a
health care professional. The publisher and author are not responsible
for any adverse effects or consequences resulting from the use of
any of the suggestions, preparations, or procedures discussed in
this book. All matters pertaining to your physical health should
be supervised by a health care professional. It is a sign of
wisdom, not cowardice, to seek a second or third opinion.

COVER DESIGNER: Jeannie Tudor
EDITOR: Michele D'Altorio
TYPESETTER: Gary A. Rosenberg

Square One Publishers
115 Herricks Road
Garden City Park, NY 11040
www.squareonepublishers.com
(516) 535-2010 • (877) 900-BOOK

ISBN: 978-0-7570-0322-6

Library of Congress Cataloging-in-Publication Data

Bruno, Gene.
  A guide to complementary treatments for diabetes / by
Gene Bruno.   p. cm.
Includes bibliographical references and index.
ISBN 978-0-7570-0322-6
1. Diabetes—Popular works. 2. Naturopathy--Popular
works. 3. Dietary supplements—Popular works. 4.
Herbs—Therapeutic use. I. Title. RC660.B78 2010
616.4'62—dc22

                              2010000494

Printed in the United States of America

10   9   8   7   6   5   4   3   2

CONTENTS

Appendices

To Uncle Frank and Uncle Phil,
whose personal struggles with diabetes
inspired me to write this book.

ACKNOWLEDGMENTS

First and foremost, I want to express my gratitude to my publisher, Rudy Shur. Not only do I appreciate his having seen the value in this book and agreeing to publish it, but further I value his skill, experience, and guidance, all of which helped me write a much better book than would otherwise have been the case.

I must also acknowledge Mel Rich, a man who inspired me and made it possible for me to pursue my education and achieve a number of professional goals. Mel, you will live forever in my heart.

My beautiful wife Kathy and my multi-talented son Jameson also deserve my thanks. Besides being my daily inspiration in life, they allowed me to use some of our precious family time to work on this book. Their love and support is the best thing that has ever happened to me.

I would be remiss if I did not acknowledge the incredibly valuable role that Cheryl Freeman has played and continues to play in my professional life. As the Director of Student Services and Registrar at Huntington College of Health Sciences, Cheryl takes care of everything and always picks up the slack when I am unable to do so. Her dedication is especially helpful when I am busy doing something, as I was when writing this book. Cheryl, there has never been a more valuable employee, and I am truly grateful for you.

I would also like to give special thanks to my friend and colleague Jennifer Hofheins, MS, RD, LD, instructor at

Huntington College of Health Sciences and Chief Operating Officer at The Center for Applied Health Sciences in Fairlawn, Ohio. Jennifer allowed me to use a menu she created and some other valuable dietary information that I have included in Appendix A of this book.

Last, but certainly not least, I thank my brilliant friend, Baron Brooks. Baron's kindness and the amazing relationships he has with so many people have helped me during an important transition in my life.

How to Use This Book

Most of the chapters in this book focus on specific complications associated with diabetes. Therefore, the book is designed in a way that readers can skip directly to the chapters that interest them or that speak to their own personal difficulties. However, I recommend that *all* readers read the first four chapters, since these are universal to anyone who has diabetes and provide valuable information for all diabetics and their families.

The various chapters of *A Guide to Complementary Treatments for Diabetes* will recommend specific therapies that readers might choose to integrate into a total diabetic healthcare program. Some of these therapies will seem familiar to some readers, but it is unlikely that any reader will recognize them all. Consequently, I prepared Appendix C, which provides an alphabetical listing and explanation of each of the complementary therapies in discussed in this book. Anytime you read about a complementary therapy that you are not familiar with, you can turn to Appendix C for an explanation.

INTRODUCTION

There are many books written on the subject of diabetes. So why write another? To me, there was only one good reason to do so: because there was something different to offer, something that has not already been said, something that can really help people. That is why I wrote *A Guide to Complementary Treatments for Diabetes*.

The vast majority of diabetes books that I have read address issues relating to dietary modification and the use of diabetic medications (like insulin). There are a few, however, that suggest if you follow the author's program it will be possible to eliminate or otherwise improve diabetes. In these cases, I have often found that the author's program focuses on some variation of dietary modification, and that the program is intended to be an alternate or replacement for the diabetic's existing diet and drug program prescribed by his or her doctor. Furthermore, these books devote relatively few pages to the use of dietary supplements and, in most cases, no pages to the use of other complementary therapies. If included at all, the pages that do discuss supplements do so in a general way and do not organize the use of supplements based upon specific diabetic complications.

A Guide to Complementary Treatments for Diabetes is different. The key word is "complementary," not "alternative." This is a book about using dietary supplements and other complementary therapies to help treat diabetes and the most common complications that arise from it. As the word complementary implies, this book is meant to be an adjunct to the patient's existing diet and drug program, *not* a replacement for that program. *A Guide to Complementary Treatments for Diabetes* assumes that readers have already received dietary instruction from their physician, nutritionist, or dietician (although Chapter 2 does provide an introductory discussion on the importance of proper diet for the diabetic, just in case).

It is my hope that this book will encourage readers to work with their doctors to utilize certain dietary supplements and complementary medicine practices to help better manage their diabetes. All the information presented is highly credible, with a solid foundation in science and references cited for all research and studies discussed. Nevertheless, the text is written in a way that anyone—regardless of their knowledge on the subject—can easily understand.

The book is separated into chapters that each explore and answer questions about a specific issue related to diabetes. Chapters 1 through 4 address basic diabetes topics that almost any diabetic can relate to, such as defining what diabetes is, the issue of dietary modification for diabetics, a basic vitamin/ mineral program that any diabetic can follow, and dietary supplements and complementary therapies that can lower blood glucose and A1C levels.

Chapters 5 through 9 cover a more broad range of issues that diabetics are prone to, but not every diabetic will experience. These include diabetic neuropathies, cardiovascular issues, circulation problems, eye issues, and weight gain. Each chapter lists dietary supplements that can aid in improving a particular issue, along with complementary treatments that can have similar results. Each supplement and therapy is generally safe for diabetics and has research and studies to back up its effectiveness and credibility.

The book is designed so that readers can simply turn to the

page of the problem they are facing, without having to read the entire book. I feel that this makes the guide more accessible. However, I recommend that everyone read Chapter 10, "How to Choose and Use Dietary Supplements." This chapter answers some common questions about dietary supplements, and in doing so provides guidelines for identifying good dietary supplements from potentially ineffective products that you do not want to waste your money on.

Happy reading!

CHAPTER 1

WHAT IS DIABETES?

Since you are reading this book, it is likely that you or a loved one has already been diagnosed with diabetes. If this is the case, you probably understand the basics of what diabetes is about. Consequently, the purpose of this chapter is not to define the disease itself, but rather to explain some of the key things you should know about this high blood glucose (blood sugar) disorder. This is so that you can learn to live with diabetes, perhaps even thrive with the disease, and—most importantly—stay healthy.

SYMPTOMS OF DIABETES

Diabetes is characterized by a variety of symptoms. If you have not been diagnosed with diabetes but think you may have it, compare the symptoms you are experiencing to the symptoms on the following list. If two or more match up, it would be a good idea to see your doctor for a proper test and diagnosis.

Common Symptoms of Diabetes

- Blurred vision
- Dehydration
- Fatigue
- Frequent urination
- Increased appetite
- Increased infections
- Increased thirst
- Weight loss

Not everyone who suffers from diabetes will experience the same symptoms. Diabetes is a disease where the sufferer has higher-than-normal blood glucose levels. A normal range for fasting blood sugar is 60 to 109 milligrams per deciliter (mg/dL). When a person's fasting blood glucose level is over 200 mg/dL, his or her kidneys lose their ability to reabsorb glucose back into the blood, causing some glucose to spill into the urine. In turn, these high glucose levels in the urine draw additional water from the blood, which increases the amount of urine produced. These people will likely experience frequent urination, dehydration, and an increased thirst. However, this is not the case for everyone. For some, constant fatigue is the only overt symptom.[1]

DIAGNOSING DIABETES

Because diabetes is characterized by high glucose levels (which result from the body's inability to make or use sufficient amounts of insulin), the diagnosis of diabetes is based primarily upon a measurement of blood glucose levels. Typically, this is done by means of a blood glucose test. A diagnosis of diabetes is made based upon the test results, which differ depending on the type of test used.

Table 1.1 shows the glucose levels that would be an indication of diabetes, depending on the blood test used.[2] Please keep in mind that a non-diabetic person could possibly have glucose levels of 200 mg/dL after eating a meal, so these blood test results are just one factor in making a diabetes diagnosis. If someone has diabetes, symptoms of the disease will be present in addition to high glucose levels.

A diagnosis of diabetes is not as straightforward as simply having the disease or not having it. There are different types of diabetes and pre-diabetes, all of which will be discussed in the next section.

Table 1.1 Glucose Levels Indicating Diabetes	
Test Type	**Glucose Levels**
Eight-Hour Fast	126 mg/dL or greater
Fasting Blood Glucose Test	200 mg/dL or greater
Random Blood Glucose Test	200 mg/dL or greater

TYPES OF DIABETES

There are three types of diabetes: type-1, type-2, and gestational.

Type-1 diabetes, previously called insulin-dependent diabetes mellitus or juvenile-onset diabetes, accounts for 5 to 10 percent of all diagnosed cases of adult diabetes. Although type-1 diabetes usually only affects children and young adults, it can occur at any age. This type of diabetes is primarily an autoimmune disease because with type-1, the body's immune system destroys beta cells in the pancreas (beta cells make insulin).

To date, no specific ways to prevent type-1 diabetes have been established. Treatment typically involves having insulin delivered by an injection or a pump. A healthy meal plan and exercise program should also be part of the treatment strategy.[3] See Chapter 2 (page 13) for more information about this.

Type-2 diabetes, previously called non-insulin-dependent diabetes mellitus or adult-onset diabetes, accounts for about 90 to 95 percent of all diagnosed cases of diabetes. Type-2 usually starts as insulin resistance, a disorder in which the cells do not use insulin effectively. Unfortunately, as the body's need for insulin increases, the pancreas gradually loses its ability to produce it.

People with type-2 diabetes can often control their blood glucose by following a healthy meal plan and exercise program, losing excess weight, and taking oral medication that helps lower glucose levels. However, some people with type-2 diabetes may also need insulin to control their blood glucose.[4] Chapter 2 (page 13) provides more information about this.

Gestational diabetes is a type of glucose intolerance that occurs during pregnancy. Women who suffer from this type of diabetes require treatment to normalize their maternal blood glucose levels. This is to avoid complications in the infant.

Immediately after the pregnancy, 5 to 10 percent of women who had gestational diabetes are found to have diabetes, usually type-2. The remaining 90 to 95 percent women who do not receive a diagnosis of diabetes immediately after delivery have a 40 to 60 percent chance of developing type-2 diabetes in the next five to ten years.[5]

Pre-Diabetes

Before people develop type-2 diabetes, they almost always have "pre-diabetes," a condition where blood glucose levels are higher than normal but not yet high enough to be diagnosed as diabetes. This may be verified with a glucose test after an overnight fast, or after a two-hour glucose tolerance test (see Table 1.2).

There are approximately 57 million people in the United States who have pre-diabetes. Recent research has shown that some long-term damage to the body, especially the heart and

Table 1.2 Glucose Levels Indicating Pre-Diabetes	
Test Type	**Glucose Levels**
Overnight Fast	100 to 125 mg/dL
Two-Hour Glucose Tolerance Test	140 to 199 mg/dL

circulatory system, may already be occurring during pre-diabetes. Research has also shown that if you take action to manage your blood glucose when you have pre-diabetes, you can delay or prevent type-2 diabetes from ever developing.

People with pre-diabetes are at increased risk of developing type-2 diabetes and heart disease, or of having a stroke.

COMPLICATIONS OF DIABETES

When blood glucose levels remain high and largely uncontrolled for a long period of time, the result can be a variety of serious complications. These complications include, but are not limited to, neuropathy (pain in the hands and feet); high blood pressure, cholesterol, and triglyceride levels; peripheral vascular disease (including pain when walking and foot ulcers); retinopathy (the leading cause of blindness worldwide); and weight gain or obesity. (Subsequent chapters are devoted to these complications, with a specific focus on which dietary supplements and complementary therapies can help treat each one.)

Many of these complications are the result of glycosylated protein (also known as glycated protein), which is protein that glucose has attached itself to. For example, glucose can attach itself to the protein in the hemoglobin in your red blood cells and form glycosylated hemoglobin, also called hemoglobin A1C, HbA1C, or just A1C for short. If this process continues, eventually you will end up with compounds called advanced glycosylation (or glycated) end products (AGEs). These AGEs become permanent fixtures in our cells.

AGEs are very reactive, frequently interacting with one another and other proteins. In the case of blood capillaries, this can result in the walls of the capillaries thickening, eventually blocking off blood vessels. This is the underlying cause of kidney complications (nephropathy) and eye complications (retinopathy).

Having high levels of cellular sorbitol (a type of sugar alcohol) may also result in diabetes complications. When you have high glucose levels, sorbitol is produced in high concentrations. Intracellular sorbitol (an accumulation of sorbitol within the cells) disrupts the pressure balance between the inside and outside of the cell, allowing water to enter the cell. The water causes the cell to swell. This process is what is believed to be— at least in part—responsible for the nerve damage (neuropathy) caused by diabetes. (Please note that this does not mean that consuming sorbitol in foods will have the same effect—it will not.)

The Importance of Blood Glucose Numbers

Research shows that keeping your blood glucose at normal levels reduces your chance of experiencing diabetic complications. To do this, you need to know your blood glucose numbers and your target goals.

There are two different tests to measure your blood glucose: the A1C test and the self-monitoring blood glucose (SMBG) test. The A1C test measures the amount of glucose that has attached to hemoglobin and measures your average blood glucose level over a period of three months. The SMBG test is self-administered. You do this test yourself using a drop of blood and a meter that measures the level of glucose in your blood at the time.

The A1C Test

You should have an A1C test done at least twice a year. The A1C test requires only a small blood sample, which can be taken at any time of the day. The A1C test is the best test to let you and your healthcare professional(s) know if your treatment plan is working over time. For most diabetics, the A1C goal is less than seven. An A1C result that is higher than seven means that you have a greater chance of diabetic complications. Conversely, lowering your A1C can improve your chances of staying healthy. If your number is seven or higher, you should talk to your healthcare professional about changing your treatment plan to bring your A1C number down. If you are pregnant, keeping your A1C at less than six will help ensure your baby is born healthy. If possible, women should plan ahead and work to get their A1C below six before getting pregnant.[6] Although you typically have blood drawn at a lab or your doctor's office for the A1C test, there are also A1C home testing devices. You and your doctor should decide if home testing is a good idea for you. If so, it is important to learn to do the test correctly and always discuss the results with your doctor.

The SMBG Test

Taking a SMBG test with a glucose meter helps determine how food, physical activity, and medicine affect your blood glucose levels. The readings can help you manage your diabetes day-by-day or even hour-by-hour. It's a good idea to keep a record of your test results and review it each time you visit your healthcare professional. To do a SMBG test, you use a tiny drop of blood and a meter to measure your blood glucose level. Be sure you know how to do the test correctly. Most new meters give results as plasma glucose rather than whole blood glucose and come with a guide that shows desirable levels. Plasma does not include the red blood cells, so there is more room for glucose to occupy this space. Be sure to set your blood glucose goals with your healthcare professionals.

Usually, self tests are done before meals, after meals, and/or at bedtime—but diabetics who use insulin usually need to test more often than those who do not take insulin. However, you should talk to your healthcare professionals to determine the specifics of when and how often you should check your blood glucose.[7] Most states have passed laws that require insurance to cover SMBG supplies and diabetes education. Check your coverage with your insurance plan. Medicare covers most of the cost of diabetes test strips, lancets (needles used to get a drop of blood), and blood glucose meters for people who have diabetes. If you are on Medicare, ask your doctor for details about coverage of the A1C test, diabetes supplies, diabetes education, and nutrition counseling.

CONCLUSION

Now that you have learned exactly what diabetes is and how a diagnosis is made, you will be able to make more informed decisions regarding your treatment. Although it may seem inconvenient and it may take awhile to get used to the regularity with which you must conduct the blood glucose tests (the SMBG in particular), it is vital that you do so. As previously stated, having the A1C test done at least twice a year is also important. Your healthcare professionals will need both the SMBG and A1C tests in order to get a complete picture of your blood glucose control. Without these tests, you won't be able to tell if your dietary, medical, supplemental, and complementary therapy efforts are paying off.

Of course, your diet plays a large roll in the progression and treatment of diabetes. To make sure that you are making the right dietary efforts, read on to the next chapter, which provides plenty of information regarding the proper diet for a diabetic.

CHAPTER 2

FOOD AND DIABETES

The power of food over diabetes is amazing. What you eat and how much you eat can make all the difference in the world regarding the stability of your blood glucose levels. Consequently, it is no surprise that a change in diet is the primary means for helping a diabetic to control his or her blood glucose levels and diabetes.

Presumably, if you are a diabetic, you've likely already received instruction on the importance of a good nutrition and diet plan. If you haven't, stop everything! You should contact your doctor, dietician, or nutritionist to make an appointment to obtain a personalized diet and exercise plan. The reason for this is that changing your diet is the first thing you need to do when you are diagnosed with diabetes. You may also want to sign up for a diabetic education program that will teach you what you need to do to care for your diabetes. Research has shown that early referral into this type of program can minimize the progression of type-2 diabetes. Specifically, patients should be educated about the progressive nature of diabetes and the importance of glucose control, with a focus on appropriate food choices and physical activity in conjunction with their anti-diabetes medication. The proof, of course, is in the pudding. In study after study, nutrition therapy in patients with diabetes has been shown to reduce A1C levels, which, as stated in Chapter 1, are the most accurate reflection of long-term blood glucose control.[1]

You should focus on making dietary and physical activity changes before you start taking dietary supplements. As the name suggests, a dietary supplement is just that: a *supplement* to the diet, not a proper substitute for eating a poor diet.

COMMON DIETARY CONCEPTS

There are a number of diet plans that can address diabetes and blood glucose control in a healthy manner. Additionally, there are diets that are *not* recommended for this purpose. This section includes an overview of some of the most well-known diet plans and their potential—or lack thereof—for helping you to achieve blood glucose control. A case will also be made for the consumption of organic foods.

Before jumping into an explanation of the diet plans, it is important to first ensure that you understand a couple of dietary concepts that find their way into more than one of these plans. The first concept is glycemic index, and the second is the type of dietary fat.

Glycemic Index (GI)

Glycemic index (GI) is a numerical system of measuring how fast a carbohydrate triggers a rise in circulating blood glucose—the higher the number, the faster the blood glucose response. A low GI food will cause a slow, small rise, while a high GI food will quickly trigger a dramatic spike (clearly not a good thing for a diabetic). In general, a GI of seventy or greater is considered high, a GI of fifty-six to sixty-nine is classified as medium, and a GI of fifty-five or less is considered low. With regard to carbohydrate foods, those with more fiber are likely to have a lower GI. This is because fiber causes food to break down more slowly in the digestive system, which also slows the absorption of any sugars the food contains. The result is a slower increase in blood glucose levels, which makes it easier for the body to metabolize since it doesn't require large amounts of insulin all at once. On the contrary, simple or refined carbohydrates—like most desserts or white bread and white pasta—break down rapidly and yield their sugars quickly, meaning they will generally be higher on the GI ranking. Table 2.1 (page 17) contains approximate GI values for some popular foods.[2] Additionally, there are a number of guidebooks that can help you identify the GI of various foods (see the recommended reading section in Appendix B, page 169).

What is most significant is the effect that a low-GI diet has on diabetics. In a review assessing the effects of low-GI diets on glucose control in people with diabetes, researchers examined 11 clinical studies involving 402 type-1 or type-2 diabetics whose diabetes were not already optimally controlled.[3] When these diabetics followed a low-GI diet, results showed a statistically significant decrease in A1C levels. Additionally, there were significantly fewer episodes of hypoglycemia (low blood sugar) in diabetics following a low-GI diet compared to those on a high-GI diet. Furthermore, the proportion of participants reporting more than fifteen episodes of hyperglycemia (high blood sugar) per month was significantly lower for those following a low-GI diet. The researchers in this review concluded that a low-GI diet can improve glucose control in diabetics without causing additional hypoglycemic episodes.

Similarly, other studies have shown that fiber-rich foods and other foods with low GIs can help keep post-meal glucose levels lower than would otherwise be the case. These foods may also improve insulin resistance and blood fat levels—an important goal for diabetics (see Chapter 6 on page 81).[4]

The importance of a low-GI diet for glucose control is further validated by population studies that showed high-GI and low-fiber diets are associated with a potential risk for developing diabetes. Conversely, the available evidence suggests that eating a diet rich in whole grain cereals and vegetables and low in refined grains, sucrose, and fructose contents (which is, essentially, a low-GI diet) is beneficial in the prevention of diabetes.[5]

Types of Dietary Fat

There are three types of dietary fat: saturated, polyunsaturated, and monounsaturated.

Chemically, a fat receives one of these three designations based upon the number of double bonds it possesses, and whether or not it is "saturated" with hydrogen atoms. However, the chemical way of explaining this can get complicated and isn't necessary for this book. To make things simpler, we will focus on the health-related features of these fats rather than their chemical attributes.

Saturated fat

Saturated fats are primarily found in animal foods, such as beef, pork, and dairy products. A vast number of studies have demonstrated that diets high in saturated fat are correlated with an increased incidence of atherosclerosis and coronary heart disease, as well as stroke.[6-8] Research has also shown that that people who consume diets high in saturated fats experience increases in their LDL cholesterol (bad cholesterol) and total cholesterol levels.[9] Since diabetics are already at higher risk for heart disease (see Chapter 6 on page 81), limiting your saturated fat intake can help lower your risk of having a heart attack or stroke. This can be done by making better, more appropriate food choices. Choosing leaner cuts of red or white meat rather than dark meat when eating poultry and choosing low or no fat dairy products are all good ways to do this.

Limiting your saturated fat intake is one of the single most important steps you can take to reduce your risk of cardio-

Table 2.1 Glycemic Index of Popular Foods

Food	GI*	Serving Size
Apple	38	1 medium (138 grams)
Baked potato	85	1 medium (173 grams)
Banana	52	1 large (156 grams)
Bean sprouts	25	1 cup (104 grams)
Bread, white	70	1 slice (30 grams)
Brown rice	55	1 cup (195 grams)
Carrot	47	1 large (72 grams)
Glucose	100	50 grams
Grapefruit	25	½ large (166 grams)
Honey	55	1 tablespoon (21 grams)
Ice cream	61	1 cup (72 grams)
Macaroni and cheese	64	1 serving (166 grams)
Oatmeal	58	1 cup (234 grams)
Orange	48	1 medium (131 grams)
Peanuts	14	4 ounces (113 grams)
Pizza	30	2 slices (260 grams)
Popcorn	72	2 cups (16 grams)
Potato chips	54	4 ounces (113 grams)
Raisins	64	1 small box (43 grams)
Rice, white	64	1 cup (186 grams)
Snickers candy bar	55	1 bar (113 grams)
Spaghetti	42	1 cup (140 grams)
Table sugar (sucrose)	68	1 tablespoon (12 grams)
Yogurt, lowfat	33	1 cup (245 grams)
Watermelon	72	1 cup (154 grams)

*GI values can be classified into three levels—low (ranging from 1 to 55), medium (ranging from 56 to 69), and high (ranging from 70 to 100).

vascular disease. Of course, this applies to everyone—but especially to diabetics.

Polyunsaturated fat

Polyunsaturated fat can be found mostly in grain products, fish and seafood (herring, salmon, mackerel, and halibut), soybeans, and fish oil. Heart-healthy omega-3 fatty acids are types of polyunsaturated fats. Omega-3 fatty acids have been shown to lower the risk of heart attacks.

Polyunsaturated fats are also protective against insulin resistance.[10] In fact, omega-3 polyunsaturated fats have clinical significance in the prevention and reversal of insulin resistance.[11] Furthermore, a diet high in polyunsaturated oleic acid, which can be easily achieved through consumption of peanuts and olive oil, can have a beneficial effect in type-2 diabetes and ultimately reverse the negative effects of inflammation observed in obesity and non-insulin dependent diabetes mellitus.[12]

Typically, polyunsaturated fats are liquid at room temperature, while saturated fats are solid (think of vegetable oil and butter, respectively). Polyunsaturated fats can be made solid, however, by forcing hydrogen atoms into them. That's exactly how margarine is made, and it is also where the term "hydrogenated fats" comes from. Unfortunately, during the hydrogenation process polyunsaturated fats are turned into trans fats (the term "trans" refers to a certain arrangement of atoms in the fat). Like saturated fats, trans fats can increase cholesterol levels and increase a diabetic's risk of developing cardiovascular disease.[13] Additionally, trans fats increase the risk of certain types of cancer.[14,15]

Monounsaturated fat

Monounsaturated fats are found in foods such as nuts and avocados. They are the main component of tea seed oil, olive oil, and canola oil. Monounsaturated fats are called "good" or "healthy" fats because they can lower your bad (LDL) cholesterol. The American Diabetes Association recommends eating more monounsaturated fats than saturated or trans fats in your diet.

Furthermore, a lower-carbohydrate/higher-monounsaturated fat diet resulted in lower plasma triglyceride (common blood fats) levels in type-1 diabetics than a higher-carbohydrate/lower-fat diet.[16]

MAJOR DIET PLANS

Now, we will take a look at the major diet plans. Although there were many plans to choose from, the ones that follow are the ones that I feel have the most research behind them to support or refute their use when dealing with diabetes.

The Mediterranean Diet

The Mediterranean Diet is based upon the diets of at least sixteen countries that border the Mediterranean Sea. Although there are many differences in culture, ethnic background, religion, economy, and agricultural production throughout these countries—which result in variations in food intake among the population groups—there is still a common Mediterranean dietary pattern.

The main components of the Mediterranean Diet are:

• Dairy products, fish, and poultry are consumed in low to moderate amounts

• Eggs are consumed no more than four times a week

• High consumption of fruits, vegetables, bread, whole grain cereals, potatoes, beans, nuts, and seeds

• Olive oil is used as an important monounsaturated fat source

- Very little amounts of red meat are consumed

- Wine is consumed in low-to-moderate amounts (equivalent to one glass of wine daily)

Consequently, this diet plan tends to be lower on the GI scale and includes a good balance of dietary fats. Research has shown that the Mediterranean Diet reduces both mortality and fatal and nonfatal heart attack rates, while providing protection against coronary heart disease.[17,18] Furthermore, the Mediterranean Diet has been shown to provide good control over blood glucose levels.[19]

The South Beach Diet

The South Beach Diet was designed by cardiologist Arthur Agatston and dietician Marie Almon as a diet plan to prevent heart disease. As its popularity increased, however, its use expanded into a means to lose weight.[20]

A primary principle of the South Beach Diet is to replace "bad carbohydrates" with "good carbohydrates" and "bad fats" with "good fats." Consequently, the South Beach Diet favors relatively unprocessed foods that are lower on the GI scale, such as vegetables, beans, and whole grains. This diet plan also eliminates trans fats, discourages saturated fats, and replaces them with foods rich in unsaturated fats and omega-3 fatty acid.

Overall, the South Beach Diet seems to be a good option for controlling blood glucose levels. It has also been shown to promote heart health and a healthy weight.[21]

Raw Food Vegetarian Diet

Although not always easy to follow, a raw food vegetarian diet may offer significant benefits for diabetics.[22] By its nature, it is lower in GI foods, lower in calories, and lower in protein (compared to non-vegetarian diets). Case reports have indicated that diabetic patients placed on a diet containing an increased percentage of raw food were able to decrease their insulin requirement. In fact, one patient had his insulin requirement reduced from sixty units per day to fifteen units per day.[23] Furthermore, long-term consumption of a low-calorie, low-protein vegan diet is associated with a lower risk for cardiovascular disease. This included the following parameters for lower risk: lower body mass index (BMI), lower plasma concentrations of lipids, lipoproteins, glucose, insulin, and C-reactive protein, as well as lower blood pressure (both systolic and diastolic) and thickness of the internal diameter of the carotid (a measure of heart disease risk).[24]

However, other research studies indicate that consuming a strictly raw food diet lowers plasma total cholesterol, triglyceride concentrations, and serum HDL cholesterol ("good" cholesterol) while increasing homocysteine concentrations.[25] Lower total cholesterol and triglyceride levels are a good thing, but a reduction in HDL cholesterol and an increase in homocysteine are not good. This is due to a vitamin B_{12} deficiency—but the deficiency could be easily offset by using a vitamin B_{12} supplement.[26]

Long-term benefits of following a raw food or vegan diet were also seen in a seventeen-year observational study of vegetarians and other health-conscious people attempting to follow a healthy diet. Results demonstrated that daily consumption of fresh fruit was associated with significantly reduced mortality from ischaemic heart disease and cerebrovascular disease.[27] Overall, the individuals in the study had a mortality rate equal to about half of that of the general population. Additionally, a twelve-week study on individuals following a raw food vegetarian diet experienced improvements in measures of mental and emotional quality of life.[28]

MyPyramid Diet Plan

On April 19, 2005, the United States Department of Agriculture (USDA) unveiled the new Food Pyramid, referred to as "MyPyramid." Those who follow MyPyramid are said to be on the MyPyramid Diet Plan. This plan was said to provide Americans with the ability to personalize their approach when choosing a healthier lifestyle, while also letting said Americans balance nutrition and exercise. At the same time, researchers discussing MyPyramid in the *Journal of the American Dietetic Association* have stated that MyPyramid is not "a therapeutic diet for any specific health condition."[29] However, the same researchers have noted that recommendations to follow MyPyramid are remarkably consistent with the various recommendations to control obesity and diabetes, heart disease and stroke, hypertension, cancer, and osteoporosis. This includes recommendations from the American Diabetes Association, the National Cholesterol Education Program, the American Heart Association, and the National Committee on High Blood Pressure. Nevertheless, there are not any specific studies validating MyPyramid as a diet plan for helping diabetics control their blood sugar levels.[30] Even so, it seems likely that the MyPyramid plan could indeed help diabetics.

The Atkins Diet

The Atkins diet, created by the late Dr. Robert Atkins, is a low-carbohydrate diet plan that is, for the most part, relatively high in fat and protein. The rationale for the lower consumption of carbohydrates in this plan is to limit the amount of glucose or sugars added to the body's metabolism. In essence, Dr. Atkins proposed that the body regularly produces insulin to convert excess carbohydrates into body fat, so excess carbohydrates must be eliminated as to not create more fat.[31]

While a number of scientific studies using the low-carbohydrate diet lend support to this approach for successful weight loss, the high-saturated fat content of this diet makes Atkins a bad idea for anyone who is at higher risk for heart disease (like diabetics).[32,33]

Before Starting Any Diet

With the exception of Atkins, if you follow one of these diets with a high degree of commitment, the results can be dramatic. Consequently, if you are using an oral medication to control your glucose levels, you should check with your doctor to see whether or not the dosage you are taking will need to be adjusted. If you are using insulin, you will be able to adjust your own dose based upon your glucose readings.

ORGANIC FOODS

Whatever diet plan you end up following, I would encourage you to choose foods that are organically grown whenever it is possible.

On its website, the USDA answers the question, "What is organic food?" in this way:

Organic food is produced by farmers who emphasize the use of renewable resources and the conservation of soil and water to enhance environmental quality for future generations. Organic meat, poultry, eggs, and dairy products come from animals that are given no antibiotics or growth hormones. Organic food is produced without using most conventional pesticides; fertilizers made with synthetic ingredients or sewage sludge; bioengineering; or ionizing radiation. Before a product can be labeled "organic," a Government-approved certifier inspects the farm where the food is grown to make sure the farmer is following all the rules necessary to meet USDA organic standards. Companies that handle or process organic food before it gets to your local supermarket or restaurant must be certified, too.[34]

Organically grown foods offer Americans a healthier alternative to conventionally-grown foods. Let us examine the evidence. On August 22, 2002, Dr. Erik Steen Kristensen of the Danish Research Centre for Organic Farming presented data on food safety from an organic perspective at the Fourteenth International Federation of Organic Agriculture Movements Congress in Victoria, Canada.

Dr. Kristensen offered the following reasons to consider organic foods:

• Discovery of animals with BSE (bovine spongiform encephalopathy), or mad cow disease

• Fewer pesticides, antibiotics, and additives than non-organic food has

• Increased occurrence of campylobacter in non-organic meat

• Increased occurrence of dioxin (an environmental pollutant) in food and fodder

• Increased occurrence of Salmonella in non-organic meat and eggs

• No toxic fungi from foods[35]

• Risk of listeria (a serious bacterial infection) from non-organic dairy products

Indeed, various data indicate that compared to conventionally-grown produce, organically-grown produce has:

- Lower levels of heavy metals

- Lower nitrate levels (less potential to cause cancer)

- Lower or zero levels of food additives (less food intolerance and cancer-causing potential)

- Higher phenol levels (which result in greater protection against cancer and cardiovascular disease)[36]

- Higher vitamin C levels[37,38]

Likewise, Dr. Kristensen presented data that compare conventional animal foods (like meat) to organic animal foods. His research stated that organic animal foods had:

- Higher levels of conjugated linoleic acid or CLA (which are preventive against cancer and arteriosclerosis)

- Higher levels of fat-soluble vitamins

- Higher levels of omega-3 fatty acids

- Higher levels of vitamin C

- Lower residues of medicines (less transfer of resistance genes to human pathogens)[39]

- Zero myotoxins (less potential problems for the liver, kidney, and nervous system)

Additionally, animal studies show higher fertility and less mortality in animals raised organically. Furthermore, studies have shown that when given a choice, animals prefer organic fodder to conventionally produced fodder. At this point, however, similar studies have not been conducted on humans. Collectively, though, all this data makes a pretty good case for recommending that the public make organic food choices whenever possible.[40,41]

CONCLUSION

As a diabetic, you already know the importance of keeping your blood glucose levels under tight control. To make this easier, you now know some dietary options for doing just that. Additionally, this chapter should have also provided you with an understanding of the importance of consuming organic foods whenever possible. With a change in diet (and the addition of exercise), you can potentially become healthy enough to stop taking one or more of your prescribed medications. It's true—the results *can* be that dramatic.

By adhering to one of the recommended diet plans in this chapter, you will experience other benefits as well. You can normalize your weight; lower your risk of heart disease, atherosclerosis, and stroke; and lower your blood pressure. You may even reduce your risk of developing certain types of cancer.

Furthermore, eating a healthy diet makes it more likely that you will be consuming a broader spectrum of important vitamins and minerals—although even then you still may not be getting enough. In the next chapter, we will discuss the use of a multivitamin and other key nutrients that can help assure diabetics that they are getting all of the nutrients they need.

CHAPTER 3

A BASIC VITAMIN/MINERAL PROGRAM FOR DIABETICS

I f you have diabetes, you may not metabolize your vitamins the same way non-diabetics do. You may actually have an increased need for certain key nutrients.[1] Consequently, it is important that you receive an adequate supply of those nutrients to help prevent deficiencies and to assure that your basic metabolic needs are being met. Additionally, some specific vitamins and minerals provide additional benefits to diabetics, beyond meeting basic metabolic needs.

In this chapter, we will examine and explain why diabetics should be using some basic dietary supplements. Then, we will discuss each vitamin and mineral mentioned, specifically highlighting, where applicable, the role these nutrients play in aiding diabetics.

THE NEED FOR DIETARY SUPPLEMENTS

According to the U.S. Department of Agriculture (USDA), only 10 percent of Americans follow a "good diet." The rest need improvement. For example, only 17 percent of the people studied consumed the recommended number of servings of fruit per day.[2] Furthermore, the same study showed that overall, Americans have failed to meet the Recommended Daily Allowance (RDA) for several key nutrients, including calcium, vitamin E, vitamin B_6, magnesium, and zinc.

27

Unfortunately, many of the people who are not eating a good diet or getting enough of key nutrients are diabetics.[3,4]

Lower Levels of Nutrients in our Diet

Just because a person is eating a "good" diet does not mean he or she is getting an adequate amount of nutrients. Research has shown that over a period of about ninety years, a 3 to 7 percent decrease in vitamin B_{12}, magnesium, zinc, and potassium levels occurred in our food supply.[5] Furthermore, studies from various sources demonstrated that growing conditions, agricultural technologies, and nutrient content of the soil can reduce nutrients in crops by as much as 20 percent.[6-12] After that, food preparations and storage methods can decrease some nutrients by as much as 30 percent.[13]

The end result is that even if people eat a good diet, it does not mean they are getting all of the nutrients they need. Supplementation with vitamins and minerals is still beneficial and necessary to assure adequate nutrient intake. As a matter of fact, due to the inadequate intake of nutrients, the *Journal of the American Medical Association* (not typically known to advocate dietary supplements) has recommended that all American adults take vitamin supplements.[14]

Diabetics and Supplementation

Many Americans do believe that they need to take supplements. National surveys indicate that 50 to 70 percent of Americans use dietary supplements.[15-17]

Some researchers recommend supplements only for diabetic patients, who may be at risk of vitamin or mineral deficiency.[18] Nevertheless, even diabetics who aren't suffering any nutritional deficiencies can benefit from supplementation. For example, research on patients with kidney disorders—50 percent of whom were diabetic—showed that vitamin supplements effectively lowered elevated homocysteine levels (a risk factor for cardio-vascular disease common in diabetics), even though the supple-mentation was not administered due to vitamin deficiencies.[19]

Given the difficulty many people have in maintaining a good diet, many healthcare professionals recommend diabet-ics take daily supplements as a form of insurance, with special consideration for key nutrients (discussed later in this chap-ter).[20] This seems to be the most sensible approach, since it guarantees diabetics will receive benefits from the nutrients, even if they are not deficient in them specifically.

IMPORTANT DIETARY CONCEPTS

Before jumping into an explanation of the nutrients diabetics should take, it is necessary to examine two important concepts that should be understood first: glycation and oxidative dam-age by free radicals.

Glycation

Although we've previously discussed the general concept of glycation, it is important to review and understand that it is a major cause of damage to various proteins in the body, and ultimately affects the tissues formed by those proteins. This process is worse with diabetes because glucose and other sugars in plasma are at increased levels. This results in advanced glycated end products (AGEs), which ultimately lead to the development of diabetic complications.[21,22] The formation of AGEs can be seriously reduced with good blood glucose control, and may be suppressed by supplementation with some nutrients.[23]

Oxidative Damage by Free Radicals

Free radicals are "chemical buzz bombs" generated as part of normal metabolism, but they can also be created through a variety of external sources. Free radicals cause oxidative damage (damage that oxygen causes to cells and DNA) that can have many negative ramifications with regard to health. Evidence indicates that free radicals generated by high blood glucose levels play a role in the development of diabetic complications. Additionally, free radicals are a root cause in the development of insulin resistance, pancreatic beta-cell dysfunction, impaired glucose tolerance, and type-2 diabetes.[24-26] A mixture of antioxidant vitamins and minerals can reduce oxidative damage caused by free radicals.[27]

IMPORTANT NUTRIENTS FOR DIABETICS

Now that we have established that diabetics can benefit from vitamins and minerals, the next obvious question is which vitamins and minerals, and how much of them?

In this section, you will find a brief description of the various vitamins and minerals diabetics can benefit from. The specific amount (or a range of amounts) diabetics should take is indicated for each nutrient.

B-Complex Vitamins

Each of the B vitamins (collectively called "B-complex vitamins") is converted into coenzymes in the body. (Coenzymes are substances that work with cellular enzymes to help facilitate their activity.) These B-vitamin coenzymes are involved, directly or indirectly, in the metabolism of energy. Some are facilitators of energy-releasing reactions; others help build new cells to deliver oxygen and nutrients that permit the energy pathways to run.

B-complex vitamins are also intimately involved in the function of the nervous system. A human's ability to respond to stresses can be influenced by his or her nutritional status—including the status of key B vitamins.[28] B vitamins have been found to be utilized rapidly in nervous-emotional stress, and to reduce the effects of stress. Additionally, they play a role in preventing heart disease (see inset below).

DOSAGE

A suggested daily dose of 50 to 75 milligrams or micrograms (depending on the vitamin) of each B vitamin (except B_6, whose dose should be 100 milligrams) is recommended to help deal with stress and low energy levels. Specifically, vitamins B_1, B_2, niacin, and pantothenic acid should be 50 to 75 milligrams, while vitamin B_{12}, folic acid, and biotin should be 50 to 75 micrograms. These dosages can be found in most high-potency multivitamin supplements.

Beta-carotene

Beta-carotene is known as "pre-vitamin A" since the body can convert it into vitamin A as needed. Beta-carotene is also an effective antioxidant. Blood concentrations of this nutri-

---

B Vitamins and Preventing Heart Disease

A substantial body of scientific evidence suggests that generous intakes of three B vitamins—B_6, B_{12}, and folic acid—may reduce the incidence of two of the primary causes of death and disability in the United States—heart disease and stroke. Scientists believe these B vitamins may reduce cardiovascular disease by lowering blood levels of homocysteine, the amino acid byproduct of metabolism. Numerous studies indicate that homocysteine levels can be effectively lowered in patients with cardiovascular disease, as well as other conditions, by using vitamin B_6, vitamin B_{12}, and folic acid, either individually or in combination.[29–37]

ent have been shown to be significantly lower in type-2 diabetic patients than in non-diabetic subjects.[38] Also, studies have shown that elderly type-2 diabetics display a significant age-related decline in blood levels of carotenoids.[39] In addition, total blood levels of antioxidants, including beta-carotene, have been shown to be significantly lower in diabetics with retinopathy (damage to the eye's retina that occurs with long-term, poorly controlled diabetes) than in diabetics who were not developing retinopathy.[40] Since the body only converts beta-carotene to vitamin A as needed, there is virtually no risk of vitamin A toxicity when supplementing with beta-carotene.

DOSAGE

Supplementation with up to 25,000 International Units (IU, see inset below) of beta-carotene daily has been proven safe and effective.

What are International Units (IU)?

While many vitamins are measured by weight in milligrams (mg) or micrograms (mcg), vitamins A, D and E are measured in International Units (IU) instead. IU is a measurement of the nutrient's activity in the body, rather than its weight. This is done because different forms of the same vitamin can have greater or lesser activity in the body. For an example, while one form of vitamin E may provide 1 IU per milligram, another form of vitamin E may provide 1 IU per 0.85 milligrams. Consequently, these vitamins are expressed on the label in IU so that consumers are provided with equivalent information about the actual vitamin potency or activity, regardless of its weight.

Calcium

Calcium is necessary for the formation of bones and teeth, blood clotting, and for normal muscle and nerve activity. Adequate calcium levels, along with regular exercise and a healthy diet, help maintain good bone health, and may help teen and young adult women reduce their high risk for osteoporosis later in life.

A review and scientific analysis of many studies has suggested that vitamin D and calcium deficiencies have a negative influence on post-meal glucose levels and insulin response, as well as an apparent relationship with type-2 diabetes.[41] Conversely, supplementation with these nutrients may be beneficial in optimizing glucose metabolism. Metformin, a medication for individuals with type-2 diabetes, decreases vitamin B_{12} absorption by tying up free calcium required for absorption of the vitamin B_{12} complex. This effect is correctable by supplementing with calcium.[42]

DOSAGE

The recommended daily dosage for calcium is 1,000 milligrams. Assuming that you're receiving some calcium from your diet, I recommend that you obtain between 500 and 600 milligrams of calcium from a supplement. A multiple mineral tablet is a good way to do this, and with the tablet you will also receive other key minerals at the same time.

Chromium

Chromium is necessary in the formation of glucose tolerance factor (GTF), a complex that works with the hormone insulin. Diabetics often have chromium levels that are below average.[43,44] In a randomized, placebo-controlled study, 180 men and women with type-2 diabetes were divided into three groups. One group was supplemented with a placebo; another with 200 micrograms of chromium daily; and the third with

1,000 micrograms of chromium daily. (For both doses, the chromium was from chromium picolinate, a well-absorbed form of this mineral).[45] Subjects continued to take their normal medications and were instructed not to change their normal eating and living habits. The results were that after two months, both doses of supplemental chromium had significant beneficial effects on A1C, glucose, insulin, and cholesterol variables.

Other studies show that taking chromium picolinate orally can decrease fasting blood glucose, A1C, and triglyceride levels, while increasing insulin sensitivity in people with type-2 diabetes.[46,47]

DOSAGE

I recommend that diabetics get at least 200 micrograms of chromium daily. However, other research shows benefits for diabetics up to 1,000 micrograms. If you'd like to try the higher dose, I recommend starting with 400 to 600 micrograms, and then increasing it by 200 micrograms at the start of each new week until you've reached 1,000. These amounts will not typically be found in a multiple mineral, and will require an additional chromium supplement.

Copper

Copper, with iron, is necessary for the formation of red blood cells and nerve fibers. It is also necessary in energy production, connective tissue formation, central nervous system function, and the formation of the hair and skin pigment melanin.

DOSAGE

Copper's recommended daily intake value of 2 milligrams is a good dose.*

---

* The "daily value" is a type of one-size-fits-all version of the RDA designed for purposes of labeling food and supplements.

Iodine

Iodine is an essential component of thyroid hormones, which regulate a number of physiological processes including growth, development, metabolism, and reproductive function.

DOSAGE

Taking 150 micrograms a day is an adequate amount for diabetics.

Iron

Iron is part of the protein hemoglobin, which carries oxygen from place to place in the body. It is also part of the protein myoglobin, which makes oxygen available for muscle contractions. Iron is necessary for the utilization of energy at a cellular level.

Some concern has been raised about a possible relationship between iron intake in men and coronary heart disease (CHD). However, a systematic review of twelve studies—including 7,800 cases of CHD—did not find sufficient evidence to support this.[48,49] Conversely, two large studies found that increased dietary heme iron (iron found in hemoglobin from animal foods such as beef) was associated with an increased risk of myocardial infarction (a heart attack). Total dietary iron was not. When stored iron levels are high, non-heme iron absorption is inhibited more effectively than heme iron absorption, suggesting that iron from animal sources may play a larger role in CHD risk than total iron does.[50] Additionally, iron may play a role in constipation (see inset on page 36).

DOSAGE

Although the relationship between iron and CHD requires further clarification, it would be prudent for adult men to avoid excess iron intake in supplements. Therefore, I suggest no more than 10 milligrams of iron per day for men, even though the

---

Iron and Constipation

High doses of iron can cause constipation. However, if you are taking less than 45 milligrams of iron a day this is unlikely—although about 10 percent of people who take iron supplements at a usual dose (18 milligrams) experience constipation anyway. The form of iron that is most frequently reported to cause constipation is ferrous sulfate. Forms of iron supplements that are less likely to cause constipation include ferrous fumarate, ferrous gluconate, heme iron concentrate, and iron glycine amino acid chelate.

---

recommended daily intake for all adults is 18 milligrams. I would say the same for postmenopausal women, who do not require as much iron as premenopausal women. Premenopausal women have a greater need for iron than men and postmenopausal women because they lose iron in blood during their menstrual periods, and are therefore at a greater risk of iron deficiency. I recommend supplementing with 18 milligrams of iron a day for premenopausal women.

According to the Food and Nutrition Board, vegetarian men and women should consume 33 milligrams of iron daily since they don't get any iron from animal proteins.[51]

Magnesium

Magnesium is necessary for normal functioning of muscle and nervous tissue. It also plays a role in the formation of bones and teeth. Magnesium metabolism is important in regulating insulin sensitivity. Unfortunately, a magnesium deficiency is common in diabetics.[52]

Studies have shown that adults and children who have higher dietary magnesium intakes are at a reduced risk of developing type-2 diabetes.[53–56] According to one analysis of studies, increasing your magnesium intake by 100 milligrams a day is associated with a 15 percent risk reduction for developing type-2 diabetes.[57]

Although it is not clear why, type-1 diabetics tend to have low magnesium levels, For these people, magnesium given orally or by injection partially overcomes the reduced magnesium levels. In one trial, insulin requirements were lower in type-1 diabetics who were given magnesium.

DOSAGE

The recommended daily value for magnesium is 400 milligrams. This amount—or even up to 600 milligrams a day—is healthy.

Manganese

Manganese activates enzymes that play important roles in the metabolism of carbohydrates, amino acids, and cholesterol. It is needed for bone formation and wound healing (an important consideration for diabetics, who do not heal wounds as easily as others). Research suggests that a low-manganese diet may result in the development of mildly abnormal glucose tolerance.[58] In addition, urinary manganese excretion tends to be slightly higher in diabetics when compared to non-diabetics.[59]

DOSAGE

A dosage of 2 milligrams of manganese a day is appropriate.

Potassium

Potassium is necessary to help maintain normal balance and pressure of body fluids and the acid-base balance of the body. It also functions in the transmission of nerve impulses and muscle contractions. An interesting consideration is that when people are inactive and not moving much, they are unable to increase their body's potassium levels through supplementa-

Table 3.1 Foods That Help Increase Potassium Intake		
Food	Serving Size	Potassium (mg)
Banana	1 medium	422
Beans, white, canned	½ cup	595
Beet greens, cooked	½ cup	655
Blackstrap molasses	1 tbsp.	498
Carrot juice	¾ cup	517
Clams, canned	3 oz.	534
Cod, Pacific, cooked	3 oz.	439
Halibut, cooked	3 oz.	490
Lima beans, cooked	½ cup	484
Potato, baked	1 potato	610
Prune juice	¾ cup	530
Rockfish, Pacific, cooked	3 oz.	442
Soybeans, green, cooked	½ cup	485
Soybeans, mature, cooked	½ cup	443
Squash, winter, cooked	½ cup	448
Sweet potato, baked	1 potato	694
Tomato paste	¼ cup	664
Tomato puree	½ cup	549
Tuna, yellowfin, cooked	3 oz.	484
Yogurt, plain, low-fat	8 oz.	531
Yogurt, plain, non-fat	8 oz.	579

Adapted from USDA National Nutrient Database for Standard Reference, Release 21 (2008)

tion. Nevertheless, supplementation with potassium has proven to modestly lower blood pressure in both people with normal blood pressure and hypertension (high blood pressure), so clearly there is a benefit.

DOSAGE

The daily value for potassium is 3,500 milligrams. Unfortunately, the FDA has placed a maximum limit on potassium in dietary supplements at 99 milligrams per dose. Because of this, potassium is the only micronutrient (vitamin or mineral) where it is not possible to achieve the daily value by supplementation— you would need to consume about thirty-five potassium tablets a day to do this, which is very unrealistic. Therefore, it is necessary to look to food sources to provide the majority of your daily dose. Choose foods from the table on the opposite page to help assure an adequate daily intake of potassium.

Selenium

Selenium functions as a constituent of the antioxidant enzyme glutathione peroxidase (GP), which detoxifies products of oxidized fats. It is found in the red blood cells. As GP, selenium has a synergistic role with other antioxidant nutrients (such as vitamins E and C), which means it enhances their activity.

DOSAGE

Selenium's daily value is 70 micrograms, although there is value in supplementing with as high as 200 micrograms. Anywhere within that range is good.

Vitamin B$_6$

Many diabetics have low blood levels of vitamin B$_6$.[60] Diabetics with neuropathy (diabetes-associated nerve damage) have particularly low levels.[61] Research has shown that a form of vitamin B_6 known as pyridoxamine can reduce the oxidative stress-induced damage associated with glycation and AGEs.[62-65]

DOSAGE

In order to reduce glycation and AGE damage, about 100 milligrams of vitamin B_6 from pyridoximine or pyridoxine hydrochloride is recommended, which is considerably higher than the 2 milligram daily value for this nutrient. This is a safe amount to use.

Vitamin C

Vitamin C has many important functions in the body, the chief ones being collagen synthesis (strengthens blood vessel walls, forms scar tissue, provides matrix for bone growth), antioxidant protection against free radicals, thyroxin synthesis, amino acid metabolism, strengthening resistance to infection, and aiding in the absorption of iron.

High blood glucose levels cause an increase in urinary loss of vitamin C. This may explain why diabetic patients are known to have low levels of vitamin C.[66,67] In addition, as with vitamin A and beta-carotene, blood levels of vitamin C have been shown to be significantly lower in diabetic patients with retinopathy than in diabetics who were not developing retinopathy.[68]

Low levels of vitamin C may make diabetics more susceptible to wound infection, delayed healing, endothelial dysfunction, and tenosynovial disease. In smokers, it may be necessary to replace the amount of vitamin C lost.[69]

For diabetics, the benefits of vitamin C supplementation include reducing glycation and lowering sorbitol levels, which is important because cellular sorbitol accumulation can damage the eyes, nerves, and kidneys of diabetics.[70,71] Also, taking a vitamin C supplementation daily for one year significantly reduced urinary protein loss in diabetics, which is important since urinary protein loss is associated with poor prognosis in diabetes.[72] This is consistent with research showing a decreased likelihood of retinopathy among diabetics taking vitamin C or E supplements, compared with those who reported no use of supplements.[73] In addition, a 16-year observational study of 85,000 women—of whom 2 percent were diabetic—found that vitamin C supplementation was associated with significant reductions in the risk of fatal and nonfatal coronary heart disease in the entire cohort.[74]

DOSAGE

While the government's daily value for vitamin C is 60 milligrams, some research indicates the optimal daily intake should be between 500 and 3,000 milligrans. I personally recommend that most diabetics use 1,000 milligrams daily.

Vitamin D

The primary role vitamin D plays in human nutrition is to facilitate the absorption of calcium and phosphorus from the intestinal tract, thereby promoting mineralization of the bones. Vitamin D is known as "the sunshine vitamin" since the ultraviolet rays of the sun can convert a cholesterol derivative in the skin into vitamin D.

People with low levels of vitamin D are at higher risk of developing insulin resistance and metabolic syndrome (prediabetes).[75] Vitamin D insufficiency or deficiency is common in diabetics, and repletion might improve glycemic control early in type-2 diabetes.[76] Research suggests that insufficient vitamin D levels may have an adverse effect on insulin secretion and glucose tolerance in type-2 diabetes.[77-79] Therefore, it is important for diabetics to supplement with vitamin D.

DOSAGE

I recommend a daily dose that is between 1,000 and 2,000 IU, which is higher than the 400 IU daily value for this nutrient. The reason for this is that new research suggests that these higher doses may be beneficial and safe for a myriad of health needs. Somewhere in this range of 400 to 1,000 IU can be achieved in a high potency multivitamin.

Vitamin E

The chief functions of vitamin E in the body are to provide antioxidant protection against free radicals, stabilize cell membranes, regulate oxidation reactions, and protect polyunsaturated fatty acids and vitamin A. Because of this, vitamin E is considered by many to be the most important of all antioxidant and cardiovascular support vitamins. Additionally, vitamin E protects red blood cells, which are important because they deliver oxygen to the body's tissues.

Some research has shown that plasma* vitamin E levels are significantly lower in subjects with poorly controlled type-2 diabetes. The same goes for subjects with type-2 diabetes that is complicated with coronary heart disease.[80] Also, elderly type-2 diabetics have shown a significant age-related decline in blood levels of vitamin E.[81] In addition, as with vitamin A, beta-carotene, and vitamin C, blood levels of vitamin E have been shown to be significantly lower in diabetic patients with retinopathy than in diabetics who were not developing retinopathy.[82]

Research conducted on type-1 diabetics suggests that daily supplementation with vitamin E for three months lowers A1C and triglyceride levels.[83]

---

* The yellow-colored liquid component of blood, in which blood cells are suspended.

DOSAGE

Studies using 300, 600, 800, and 1,200 IU doses of vitamin E in diabetics have also shown a reduction in glycation.[84-86] I suggest 400 IU daily for most diabetics, but those with a history of heart disease may wish to increase the dose.

Vitamin K

Vitamin K is essential for the functioning of several proteins involved in blood clotting.[87] In addition, vitamin-K dependent proteins are necessary for bone mineralization (helping to keep calcium in the bone).[88]

There are two naturally occurring forms of vitamin K. Plants synthesize phylloquinone, which is also known as vitamin K_1. Bacteria synthesize a range of vitamin K forms collectively referred to as vitamin K_2.[89]

A vitamin K deficiency is uncommon in healthy adults. Elderly diabetics, however, may be at risk for drug-induced vitamin K deficiency.[90] Another consideration is that vitamin K antagonizes the effects of oral anticoagulants such as warfarin (*Coumadin*), which may be used by some diabetics with certain cardiovascular disorders. Consequently, vitamin K is not as frequently included in multivitamins as are other nutrients.

DOSAGE

Due to the complications described, I do not usually recommend supplementation with vitamin K, unless there is an established vitamin K deficiency or a risk of osteoporosis. In that instance, the daily value dose of 80 micrograms is acceptable, although doses up to 45 milligrams daily may be used under a doctor's supervision.

Zinc

Zinc is a versatile trace mineral required as a cofactor by hundreds of enzymes in every organ of the body. It is also associated with the hormone insulin. Zinc is involved in making genetic material and proteins, immune reactions, transporting vitamin A, taste perception, wound healing (an important consideration for diabetics), making sperm, and the normal development of the fetus.

Men with low zinc intake may experience reduced levels of serum testosterone concentrations and the volume of semen they ejaculate. In addition, seminal loss also accounts for 9 percent of total body zinc loss when the individual has low zinc intake. Furthermore, some men lose significantly more zinc in their semen than others. Since men lose zinc every time they ejaculate, supplementation with zinc may help to assure adequate replenishment of this mineral.

DOSAGE

For men, a daily dose of 25 milligrams of zinc is recommended. Due to the reasons previously stated, this is higher than the daily value of 15 milligrams. For women, 15 milligrams is just fine.

Other Nutrients: Phosphorus, Sodium, and Chloride

Phosphorus, sodium, and chloride are all important minerals that play vital functions in human health. However, it is generally not necessary to supplement with them for one simple reason: Americans already consume adequate or excessive amounts of these minerals.

For example, diets that provide adequate calories and protein also supply adequate phosphorus. Dietary deficiencies of phosphorus are unknown. Animal protein is a rich source of phosphorus. Additionally, phosphorus from additives in processed foods can significantly add to people's intakes.[91]

In the case of sodium and chloride, both of these minerals can be found in common table salt, which people often consume in excessive quantities.[92]

A BASIC FOUNDATION PROGRAM

While reading about the various nutrients in this chapter, you may have thought you would have to swallow handfuls of pills to meet all of the recommendations being made. Luckily, that is not what is needed. Instead, most of the nutrients in the doses recommended can be achieved by using a basic foundation program (BFP). Many individuals wrongly assume that a single multivitamin product will provide this. However, unless the multivitamin were the size of a golf ball, it would be unable to provide optimal doses of each vitamin and mineral.

A more realistic approach is to obtain optimal doses from four dietary supplements: a multivitamin, a vitamin C product, a vitamin E product, and a multiple-mineral product.

The following are guidelines that you can use while shopping for these products.

Multivitamin

A multivitamin is a capsule or tablet containing doses of more than one vitamin. A good multivitamin should provide adequate doses of the B-vitamins, vitamin A, and vitamin D.

Other nutrients such as vitamin C, E, and minerals will be present, but at suboptimal doses.

Multivitamin Tips

The B-complex and vitamin C are water-soluble vitamins. Since the body doesn't really store water soluble vitamins (with the exception of vitamin B_{12}), any vitamin that hasn't been used within one to three hours after ingestion will be excreted. Therefore, it is a good idea to get a multivitamin that is time-released since the vitamin may be released over a period of 8 to 12 hours. Research has indicated that while 30 percent of vitamin C from a regular tablet is excreted into the urine, only 14 percent of vitamin C is excreted from a time-released tablet.[93] Time-releasing may cost a little more, but your body will use more of the vitamins and excrete less of them.

The following chart lists the nutrients a good multivitamin should contain, and provides appropriate amounts for each nutrient.

Nutrient	Recommended Dosage
Biotin	50 to 75 micrograms
Folic acid	100 to 400 micrograms
Niacin/Niacinamide	50 to 75 milligrams
Pantothenic acid	50 to 75 milligrams
Vitamin A/Beta-carotene	10,000 to 25,000 IU
Vitamin B_1	50 to 75 milligrams
Vitamin B_2	50 to 75 milligrams
Vitamin B_6	50 to 100 milligrams
Vitamin B_{12}	50 to 75 micrograms
Vitamin D	400 to 2,000 IU

Vitamin C

When shopping for vitamin C at your vitamin or health food store or online retailer, be sure to check the information on the following chart to ensure it matches with the product you choose:

Nutrient	Recommended Dosage
Bioflavonoids	250 to 500 milligrams
Vitamin C	1,000 milligrams

Vitamin C Tips

Your body can easily use up to 3,000 milligrams of vitamin C daily. If you are ill, your body uses even more than this. As with multivitamins, vitamin C should also be time-released.

It is a good idea to look for a vitamin C product that contains bioflavonoids (or flavonoids), which are substances found wherever vitamin C is found in nature—essentially, in a variety of fruits and vegetables. Bioflavonoids have been shown to improve the therapeutic action of vitamin C. They help keep vitamin C in its active, antioxidant form rather than its inactive, oxidative form.[94]

Vitamin E

When shopping for a vitamin E product, be sure to check the information on the following chart to ensure it matches with the product you choose:

Nutrient	Recommended Dosage
Vitamin E (d-alpha)	400 IU

Additional beta, delta, and gamma tocopherols (which are other forms of vitamin E) or tocotrienols (which are vitamin E relatives with antioxidant properties) are a plus.

Vitamin E tips

Natural vitamin E is better than synthetic vitamin E. In fact, research has shown that natural vitamin E is 3.5 times more active in the human body than synthetic vitamin E, even though the same number of IUs of natural and synthetic were used for the study.[95] Therefore, you should always use natural vitamin E rather than the synthetic version. You can tell the difference because natural vitamin E is designated as "d-alpha" tocopherol/tocopheryl, while synthetic vitamin E is designated as "dl-alpha". When you see the "l" after the "d," the product is synthetic.

Multiple Mineral

A good multi-mineral supplement will provide about 50 to 100 percent of the daily value for all of the minerals you see listed in the following chart:

Nutrient	Recommended Dosage
Calcium	500 to 600 milligrams
Chromium	25 to 100 micrograms
Copper	1 to 2 milligrams
Iodine	75 to 150 micrograms
Iron	10 to 18 milligrams
Magnesium	250 to 300 milligrams
Manganese	2 milligrams
Potassium	50 to 99 milligrams
Selenium	25 to 100 micrograms

When shopping for a multiple mineral, try to get one that mataches (or comes close to matching) the dosages in the chart.

Multiple Mineral Tips

Minerals can be chelated to improve their absorption. Chelation is a term that refers to attaching an organic acid (such as an amino acid) to a mineral element. For example, if you attached citric acid to calcium, you would have a chelated form of calcium called calcium citrate. Calcium citrate has been shown to have about a 13 percent greater calcium absorption than the commonly used form of calcium carbonate.

The problem with chelated minerals is that they generally provide less of the mineral element and more of the chelating agent. Let's examine calcium citrate, which provides about 22 percent actual or elemental calcium. By comparison, calcium carbonate provides about 38 to 40 percent elemental calcium.

The bottom line is that while chelated minerals are better absorbed than common mineral forms, what is most important is to get the correct elemental amount of the mineral—and chelated minerals are not always the best way to do this. Make sure to take the mineral supplement with a meal so that the hydrochloric acid in your stomach will break it down efficiently for absorption.

CONCLUSION

If you are a diabetic, you should be taking dietary supplements because the chances are you are not getting sufficient amounts of all the nutrients you need by diet alone. Furthermore, various key nutrients may provide you with additional benefits and help to reduce your risk of certain deficiencies. Optimal levels of these key nutrients can be obtained in a basic foundation program consisting of a multiple vitamin, a vitamin C, a vitamin E, and a multiple mineral. Regular use of a basic foundation program will support the health and well-being of diabetics, and may even play a role in the prevention of some diabetic complications.

In the next chapter, we will focus on blood glucose control, which is the very best thing we can do to reduce diabetic complications.

CHAPTER 4

CONTROLLING
BLOOD GLUCOSE LEVELS

Even though researchers have not yet discovered a cure for diabetes, they have found effective ways to help you control your blood glucose levels. As discussed in Chapter 1, keeping your blood glucose below certain levels will help you to prevent most—if not all—of the health risks associated with diabetes.

This chapter is designed to help you understand which dietary supplements and complementary medicine practices can be used along with diet and exercise to help keep glucose levels within a normal, healthy range.

DIETARY SUPPLEMENTS

There are several dietary supplements that have the potential to help reduce blood glucose and A1C levels in diabetics. Remember, the A1C test measures the amount of glucose that has attached to hemoglobin and measures your average blood glucose over a period of three months. Some of the most effective supplements are alpha lipoic acid, biotin, chromium, cinnamon extract, Gymnema extract, milk thistle extract, Panax ginseng, and Pycnogenol, all of which will be elaborated on in this section.

Most studies on these supplements were conducted on type-2 diabetics, though some were also conducted on type-1.

In any case, given the mechanism of actions for these supplements, I tend to believe they would all be beneficial for either type-1 or type-2 diabetics.

Alpha-Lipoic Acid

Alpha-lipoic acid (ALA) is a natural antioxidant manufactured by the body. It was identified as a vitamin when it was isolated fifty years ago, but was reclassified upon the finding that it is synthesized in humans and animals.[1] Unlike most other antioxidants, however, it has the advantage of being soluble in both fat and water, so it can provide protection both inside and outside of cells.[2] ALA is also found in some foods, particularly liver and yeast.

In a placebo-controlled, multicenter study, seventy-four patients with type-2 diabetes were given either a placebo or 1,800 milligrams of ALA daily.[3] When compared to the placebo group, the people receiving the ALA had significantly greater insulin-sensitivity (reflecting improvement in insulin resistance) and reduced glucose levels. In other research, oral or intravenous use of ALA improved insulin sensitivity and reduced glucose levels in patients with type-2 diabetes.[4-6] However, some people who used ALA orally reported a skin rash.[7]

Theoretically, if you use ALA with other drugs that lower blood glucose levels (hypoglycemic agents) it might cause additional blood glucose lowering effects.[8]

DOSAGE

In these studies, patients who took a daily dose between 600 and 1,800 milligrams of ALA orally or 500 to 1,000 milligrams intravenously had significant improvement in insulin resistance and glucose effectiveness. These effects were seen after four weeks for those taking ALA orally, and after one to ten days for those using intravenous administration.

Biotin

Biotin is a B vitamin that plays various important functions, including helping the body form glucose from sources other than carbohydrates. Research has shown that a combination of biotin and chromium may lower blood glucose and A1C levels in type-2 diabetes patients. In a randomized, double-blind, placebo-controlled study, 447 subjects with poorly controlled type-2 diabetes received either 600 micrograms of chromium (from chromium picolinate) and 2 milligrams of biotin, or a placebo every day for ninety days, in combination with stable oral anti-diabetic agents.[9] Results showed a significant reduction in A1C and fasting glucose levels for those who took the supplement compared to those who took the placebo. Similar results were achieved through other studies.[10]

Biotin alone, however, does not seem to affect glucose or insulin levels in people with type-2 diabetes—only when it is combined with chromium.[11]

DOSAGE

The recommended dose of biotin is 2 milligrams (2,000 micrograms) taken with at least 600 micrograms of chromium (from chromium picolinate). However, doses of 10 milligrams per day have been taken without adverse effects. Biotin has no known interactions with drugs.

Chromium

Chromium is an essential trace mineral that works with insulin to help transport glucose throughout the body in order to maintain healthy glucose levels. Chromium levels can be below normal in patients with diabetes.[12,13]

In a randomized, placebo-controlled study, 180 men and women with type-2 diabetes were divided into 3 groups. One group was supplemented with a placebo, another with 200 micrograms of chromium per day, and the third with 1,000 micrograms of chromium per day for four months (from chromium picolinate for both doses).[14] Subjects continued to take their normal medications and were instructed not to change their normal eating and living habits for the duration of the study. The results showed that both doses of supplemental chromium had significant beneficial effects on A1C, glucose, insulin, and cholesterol levels. The benefits were greater with the higher dose.

Other studies have shown that taking chromium picolinate orally can decrease fasting blood glucose levels, decrease A1C levels, decrease triglyceride levels, and increase insulin sensitivity in people with type-2 diabetes.[15,16] Some evidence also suggests that chromium picolinate might decrease weight gain and fat accumulation in type-2 diabetics who are taking a sulfonylurea (an antidiabetic drug that acts by increasing insulin release from the beta cells in the pancreas).[17]

DOSAGE

Higher chromium doses (1,000 micrograms per day) might be more effective and work more quickly.[18] Higher doses might also reduce triglyceride and total serum cholesterol levels in some patients.[19,20] Additional research demonstrated that chromium picolinate also improved glucose levels in patients with type-1 diabetes, as well as those with gestational and steroid-induced diabetes.[21–24]

Theoretically, using chromium with other blood glucose-lowering drugs might cause additional blood glucose lowering effects.[25] Taking 1,000 micrograms of chromium picolinate with 1 milligram levothyroxine per day has been shown to decrease serum levels of levothyroxine by 17 percent, when compared to taking levothyroxine alone.[26] Levothyroxine should be taken at least 30 minutes before or 3 to 4 hours after taking chromium.

For type-2 diabetics, 600 to 1,000 micrograms per day are recommended.

Cinnamon Extract

The smell and taste of cinnamon in a warm, gooey cinnamon bun is probably enjoyable to just about anyone. Unfortunately, the gooey cinnamon bun is not a particularly good choice for diabetics, but the cinnamon itself may actually provide some significant health benefits.

The majority of clinical research on cinnamon shows that whole cinnamon powder is not effective for type-1 or type-2 diabetes. However, two studies conducted on a specific water-soluble cinnamon extract both showed consistent, beneficial results.[27] A placebo-controlled, double-blind study was conducted on seventy-nine patients with type-2 diabetes.[28] Subjects were given 336 milligrams of a water-soluble cinnamon extract (corresponding to 3 grams of whole cinnamon powder) or a placebo every day for four months. Those taking the cinnamon experienced a significant 10.3 percent reduction in fasting blood sugar levels, compared to a non-significant 3.4 percent reduction in the placebo group.

In another placebo-controlled, double-blind study, twenty-one adults with metabolic syndrome (i.e., prediabetes) were given a water-soluble cinnamon extract (500 milligrams per day) or a placebo for twelve weeks.[29] The results showed that 83 percent of those given the extract experienced a significant decrease (about 8 percent) in fasting blood sugar, compared to only 33 percent of the placebo group. In addition, the subjects who took the cinnamon also experienced a significant alteration in body composition. Their body fat decreased by .7 percent, and their muscle mass increased by 1.1 percent. These changes took place without alterations in the diets or physical activity levels of the subjects.

Orally, cinnamon (in any form) appears to be well-tolerated.

DOSAGE

A good dose is 500 milligrams daily of a water-soluble cinnamon extract.

Gymnema Extract

Gymnema is an Ayurvedic (or East Indian) herb with a long history of use for treating diabetes. In an open-label study, twenty-two type-2 diabetic patients received 400 milligrams of Gymnema extract daily for eighteen to twenty months, as a supplement to the conventional oral drugs that lower blood sugar levels.[30] Subjects showed a significant reduction in blood glucose, A1C levels, and other glycosylated blood proteins. In addition, the subjects' conventional drug dosage could be decreased. Five of the twenty-two subjects were able to discontinue using their conventional drug because they could maintain their blood glucose homeostasis with Gymnema extract alone. The researchers suggested that the results may have been due to beta cell (the cells in the pancreas that are supposed to produce insulin) regeneration and/or repair, as supported by the appearance of raised insulin levels in the serum of patients after supplementation.

In a similar study, the same dose of Gymnema extract was administered to twenty-seven patients with type-1 diabetes. All the test subjects were also on insulin therapy.[31] The results showed that insulin requirements came down, together with blood glucose, A1C levels, and glycosylated blood protein levels. Blood fats also returned to near-normal levels with Gymnema therapy. The type-1 diabetic control subjects who received insulin alone without any Gymnema showed no significant reduction in serum lipids, A1C levels, or glycosylated blood protein when followed up after ten to twelve months. There were no reported adverse reactions.

In essence, what the studies showed was that Gymnema can enhance the blood glucose-lowering effects of insulin and hypoglycemic drugs.

DOSAGE

A good daily dose is 400 milligrams of Gymnema extract, standardized for 25 percent gymnemic acids.

Milk Thistle Extract

Milk thistle is, arguably, the best herbal medicine for liver health. The active components in milk thistle are its flavonoids, collectively called silymarin. The majority of milk thistle-related research has been conducted on silymarin. Silymarin has primarily been studied and recognized for its benefits to people with liver disorders, although it has benefits for diabetics as well. Studies show that taking 600 milligrams of silymarin daily for four months—in combination with conventional treatment—can significantly decrease fasting blood glucose, A1C levels, total cholesterol, low-density lipoprotein (LDL) cholesterol, and triglycerides in patients with type-2 diabetes.[32] Other research has shown that the same dose of silymarin daily (600 milligrams) reduced insulin resistance in people with coexisting diabetes and alcoholic cirrhosis.[33]

Orally, milk thistle is usually well-tolerated, but it can cause an occasional laxative effect. There are no established interactions with drugs.

DOSAGE

Using 750 milligrams of a typical milk thistle extract standardized for 80 percent silymarin would yield 600 milligrams of silymarin. This is a good daily dose.

Panax Ginseng

In Asian countries, the fleshy root of the Panax ginseng plant is considered a tonic, stimulant, and stress adaptogen (adaptogens usually exert no specific biological effects, but tend to normalize general adverse conditions of the body). More than 500 studies have been published on ginseng.

Perhaps the best known of ginseng's major properties is its ability to improve mental performance, physical performance, and wellbeing in a variety of circumstances.

In addition, this classic herbal medicine has benefits for diabetics. In a double-blind, placebo-controlled study, thirty-six type-2 diabetics were treated for eight weeks with ginseng (100 or 200 milligrams) or a placebo. The results showed that all doses of ginseng therapy improved mood and mental and physical performance, and reduced fasting blood glucose and body weight. The 200 milligram dose of ginseng improved A1C levels and physical activity. The placebo reduced body weight and altered the serum lipid profile, but did not alter fasting blood glucose.[34] Likewise, in a twelve-week, double-blind, randomized, crossover study, nineteen type-2 diabetics were supplemented with 6 grams of Panax ginseng as an adjunct to their usual anti-diabetic therapy (diet and/or medications). The results were that good blood glucose control was maintained throughout, and fasting glucose levels were reduced while fasting insulin levels were increased.[35] Since diabetics have glucose levels that are too high and insulin levels that are too low, you can see why this would be a good benefit.

Orally, Panax ginseng is usually well-tolerated. Theoretically, concurrent use with anti-diabetic drugs might enhance blood glucose lowering effects.[36] Also theoretically, concurrent use might interfere with immunosuppressive therapy since Panax ginseng might have immune system-stimulating properties.[37]

DOSAGE

A daily dose between 100 and 200 milligrams of Panax ginseng extract—providing about 7 percent of ginsenosides (active compounds in ginseng)—is a good amount.

Pycnogenol

Pycnogenol is the trade name of a bioflavonoid (the most common group of polyphenolic compounds in the human diet and found ubiquitously in plants) derived from the bark and needles of the pine tree Pinus maritima. This patented bioflavonoid contains the powerful group of antioxidants called oligomeric proanthocyanidins (OPCs). As antioxidants, OPCs are 50 times more effective than vitamin E and 20 times as strong as vitamin C (which does *not* mean that they can substitute for vitamin E and C or their antioxidant functions).

In addition, Pycnogenol may have benefits for diabetics. In an open, controlled, dose-finding study, thirty type-2 diabetics were given 50, 100, 200, and 300 milligrams of Pycnogenol daily in three-week intervals for a total of twelve weeks.[38] The doses between 100 and 300 milligrams lowered fasting glucose levels significantly, while the 50 milligram dose significantly lowered glucose levels only after a meal. The 300 milligram dose had no stronger effect than the 200 milligram dose. A1C levels decreased continuously with all doses, but a more significant difference was shown with the 200 and 300 milligram doses.

Similarly, a double-blind, placebo-controlled, randomized, multi-center study was performed with seventy-seven type-2 diabetics. The subjects were given either a placebo or 100 milligrams of Pycnogenol for twelve weeks, during which standard anti-diabetic treatment was continued. The results showed that the Pycnogenol significantly lowered plasma glucose levels as compared to the placebo. A1C levels were also lowered, although the difference when compared to placebo was statistically significant only for the first month.[39] Pycnogenol is well-tolerated. Theoretically, Pycnogenol may interfere with immunosuppressant therapy because of its immunostimulating activity.

DOSAGE

A daily dose of 100 to 200 milligrams of Pycnogenol is appropriate.

The supplements discussed in this section are not the only dietary supplements that have the potential to reduce glucose and A1C levels in diabetics. They are, however, the ones that seem to have the most data to support their use, as well as the least adverse known effects or interactions. Certain other supplements that are popular for this purpose sometimes lack good research to substantiate their use; or their potential adverse effects tend to make them too risky for diabetics.

COMPLEMENTARY TREATMENTS

In addition to dietary supplements, a number of complementary treatments exist for helping to lower blood glucose levels. As you read this section, pay special attention to the fact that some complementary treatments are good for type-1 diabetes, while others are good for type-2. Understanding this will help you focus on the type of complementary treatment(s) best able to benefit you.

Exercise

Data from twenty studies present a consistent picture indicating that regular physical activity substantially reduces the risk of developing type-2 diabetes.[40] In fact, a high level of physical activity (more than 150 minutes per week) is associated with a 20 to 30 percent reduction in diabetes risk. Clearly, this good news for those who have not yet developed diabetes. But you may be wondering: what does this mean for the people who already have it?

Lifestyle intervention programs that include exercise and healthy diets have long been known to exert beneficial effects on whole-body metabolism, in particular leading to enhanced insulin-sensitivity in type-2 diabetics.[41] In fact, in a review of twenty studies, resistance training (like weight lifting) was shown to help improve blood glucose control and insulin sensitivity in adults with type-2 diabetes. Specifically, supervised resistance training was found to provide these benefits. When supervision was removed, however, the diabetics did not tend to be as regular with their exercise, and blood glucose control decreased.[42] The take home message is that if you regularly perform resistance training (for about 20 to 30 minutes, three times a week), you are likely to experience significant benefits.

In another study, diabetic patients were randomly assigned to either supervised endurance and resistance training—four times a week for twenty-four months—or standard treatment for diabetes.[43] The results showed that maximum oxygen consumption, muscle strength, and A1C levels improved significantly for those in the exercise group, but no change or worsening in these variables occurred in the standard treatment group.

As mentioned in Chapter 3, free radicals and the oxidative damage they cause may contribute to diabetic complications. Interestingly, research has shown that there are three ways in which both short-term and long-term exercise may help reduce the oxidative stress that takes place after a meal.

• Exercise stimulates an increase in the production of anti-oxidant enzyme activity by the body, which in turn reduces oxidation.

• Exercise helps reduce blood glucose levels and enhances insulin sensitivity, which means there is less glucose to oxidize.

• Exercise improves the reduction of blood triglycerides, which means there are less triglycerides to oxidize.[44]

While exercise positively influences diabetes—including blood glucose concentrations, insulin action, and cardiovascular risk factors—diabetics should be aware that exercising does still come at a certain risk. Particularly, it can lead to low blood glucose levels (hypoglycemia). To decrease the risk of hypoglycemia, insulin doses should be reduced prior to exercise, although some insulin is typically still needed. You should talk to your doctor to determine an appropriate reduction.

Nevertheless, for patients with diabetes, the overall benefits of exercise are clearly significant. Patients should work together with their doctors to maximize these benefits while minimizing risks for negative consequences.[45]

Hypnosis

Hypnosis has a history of helping people with lifestyle changes, including eating disorders and smoking cessation.[46] It has been reported that about 20 percent of the time, adolescents with type-1 diabetes do not adhere to diet and exercise programs, as well as other self-care behaviors.[47] In a hypnosis study, six type-1 diabetic adolescents were tracked for six months. No changes were made in their insulin dose, diet, or exercise regimes.[48] Then, hypnosis was individually administered to the usual diabetes care program for six months. The results showed that average A1C levels dropped from 13.2 percent to 9.7 percent, and average fasting blood glucose (FBG) dropped from 426 mg/dL to 149 mg/dL.

Relaxation Techniques

Feeling stressed can raise blood glucose levels in diabetics due to an increased production of the stress hormones, which reduce insulin action.[49] Keeping excess stress hormones in check with relaxation and biofeedback techniques may help stabilize glucose levels and, at the same time, provide some protection for the heart, both very important issues for people with diabetes.[50] Furthermore, when in a relaxed state, the body metabolizes carbohydrates more efficiently, thereby lowering blood glucose levels.[51,52]

In dozens of published studies about diabetes and blood glucose, the most common complementary treatment is relaxation training, or biofeedback-assisted relaxation training.[53] These studies, which used biofeedback-assisted relaxation training with type-1 diabetic patients, showed a significant reduction in blood glucose levels.[54-56] As a matter of fact, type-1 diabetics have the potential to develop blood glucose levels that are a bit *too* low following relaxation, and therefore need to be prepared to compensate if necessary.[57,58]

In similar studies on type-2 diabetics, however, no significant reduction of blood glucose levels was revealed.[59,60] Nevertheless, with relaxation training, type-2 diabetics may experience other benefits, including increased self-management abilities, improved sense of well-being, increased coping skills, lowered incidence of depression, and less perceived stress.[61]

Yoga

Yoga, or Hatha yoga, is a form of meditative exercise from India that is associated with certain postures, called "asanas." A review of scientific literature has shown that yoga-based therapy for the management of type-2 diabetes has positive short-term effects on multiple diabetes-related outcomes. These include significant reductions in fasting and postprandial blood glucose levels, hemoglobin A1C, total cholesterol and low-density lipoprotein, triglycerides, oxidative stress, blood pressure, body weight, heart rate, need for medication, and psychosocial risk factors. Yoga is also associated with decreased weight gain in healthy adults, a matter of significance in the prevention and management of some chronic illnesses, including diabetes.[62] Furthermore, research has shown that Hatha yoga (physical movements and postures) and meditation (a mental discipline by which one attempts to get beyond the reflexive, "thinking" mind into a deeper state of relaxation or awareness) provide real benefits in stabilizing blood glucose.[63] A group of researchers studied the response yoga therapy had on people with type-2 diabetes. The results showed that 70 percent of participants had a fair-to-good response. After forty days, there was a significant reduction in high blood glucose levels.[64]

In a review of twenty-five studies on yoga, results suggest that doing yoga can result in beneficial changes in several diabetes risk areas, including glucose levels, insulin sensitivity, blood fat levels, blood pressure, oxidative stress, nervous system function, and lung function.[65]

Additionally, it has been suggested by some that since yoga is a simple and economical therapy, it might be considered a beneficial complementary and self-administered therapy to other medical treatment for diabetes.[66]

MONITORING YOUR GLUCOSE LEVELS

If you are currently using insulin—and you intend to start any of the supplements or programs described in this chapter—it is important to understand that these regimens will likely have an effect on the amount of insulin your body will require.

If you are using insulin, changing the amount you take will not be too hard to do since you will be testing your blood glucose before determining the appropriate insulin dose. Clearly, if your blood glucose levels are lower, you will not need as much insulin. However, this becomes more problematic if you are using an oral hypoglycemic medication, because you cannot really adjust the amount of a pill that you are swallowing. In this instance, it is particularly important that you work closely with your doctor so that adjustments can be made to your medication accordingly.

Likewise, should you have questions about using any of the above approaches, please talk to your doctor about your concerns.

CONCLUSION

Incorporating just a few of the supplementary or therapeutic suggestions in this chapter into your lifestyle can have a profound effect on your health. The ramifications of lowering and controlling high blood glucose levels are all positive. Besides a better quality of life in general, you will be far less likely to suffer from any of the other diabetic complications addressed in this book.

Nevertheless, if you are already developing (or have developed) one or more diabetic complications, the subsequent chapters may help you understand more about those complications and what you can do to make a difference. The first complication we will examine is diabetic neuropathy.

CHAPTER 5

DIABETIC NEUROPATHIES

About 60 to 70 percent of all diabetics have some form of nerve damage—a diabetic neuropathy (or, more accurately, neuropathies, since there are more than one kind). Having high blood sugar levels over a long period of time damages nerves throughout the body, but the nerves in the hands and feet are the ones most often damaged.

Symptoms of diabetic neuropathy (DN) can include pain and numbness—particularly in the hands and feet—or problems with digestion, the urinary tract, the blood vessels, or the heart. The severity of these symptoms can range between mild and extremely painful, sometimes to the point of disability.

The chapter will begin by providing some introductory information about diabetic neuropathies. Next, it will present a look at some specific dietary supplements that may help in the treatment of this problem. Finally, complementary treatments that have been shown to be beneficial for diabetic neuropathies will be discussed.

TYPES OF DIABETIC NEUROPATHIES

According to the National Institutes of Health, DNs are most common in diabetics who have problems controlling their blood glucose levels, diabetics with high blood lipid levels (high cholesterol and triglycerides), diabetics with high blood pressure, and diabetics who are overweight.[1] However, there are other factors that can contribute to the development of DNs. These other factors may include low levels of insulin, factors leading to damage to the blood vessels that carry oxygen and nutrients to nerves, autoimmune factors that cause inflammation in nerves, mechanical injury to nerves (such as carpal tunnel syndrome), inherited traits that increase susceptibility to nerve disease, and/or lifestyle factors (such as smoking or alcohol use.) The risk of developing a DN increases with age and with the length of time the individual has had diabetes. Those who have had diabetes for at least twenty-five years have the highest rates of developing neuropathy.

There are four different types of DNs, each with its own characteristics and symptoms.[2]

• Autonomic neuropathies. With autonomic neuropathies, the most common symptoms are changes in digestion, bowel function, bladder function, sexual response, and perspiration. Additionally, the nerves that serve the heart, control blood pressure, and the nerves in the lungs and eyes may be affected as well. Hypoglycemia unawareness—a condition in which people no longer experience the warning symptoms of low blood glucose levels—may also occur.

• Focal neuropathy. Focal neuropathy is classified by a sudden weakness of one nerve or a group of nerves. With focal neuropathy, any nerve in the body can be affected.

• Peripheral neuropathy. Peripheral neuropathy is the most common type of DN. It causes pain or loss of feeling in any or all of the following: toes, feet, legs, hands, and/or arms.

• Proximal neuropathy. Proximal neuropathy results in thigh, hip, or buttocks pain, and can lead to weakness in the legs.

DIETARY SUPPLEMENTS

There are a number of dietary supplements with potential to help treat DNs. Some of the most promising are acetyl-L-carnitine, alpha lipoic acid, benfotiamin, gamma linolenic acid, and methylcobalamin. This section will include a discussion of each of these supplements, along with suggested dosage information.

Acetyl-L-Carnitine

Acetyl-L-carnitine (ALC) is a form of the amino acid L-carnitine. Both help to transport fat into muscle cells, where it can be burned for energy. Additionally, ALC helps produce acetylcholine, a brain chemical that is required for various mental functions. ALC occurs naturally in the brain, liver, and kidneys.

Studies have shown that ALC levels are deficient in diabetics.[3] Results from double-blind research showed that type-1 or type-2 diabetics with peripheral neuropathy experienced improved symptoms after taking 1,500 to 3,000 milligrams of ALC daily in divided doses (two or three times a day instead of all at once) for one year. ALC seems to increase nerve fibers, regenerate clusters of nerve fibers, and improve sensations. With patients who reported pain as their most significant symptom, research showed that taking 1,000 milligrams of ALC two to three times a day decreased neuropathy-related pain within six months of beginning treatment. Lower doses (500 milligrams three times a day) did not seem to reduce pain.

According to studies, supplementation with ALC is more likely to be effective for reducing pain in patients with a shorter duration of diabetes and in patients with poorly-controlled type-2 diabetes.[4-7]

When taken orally, ALC is generally well tolerated. Taking 1 gram of L-carnitine daily has been shown to significantly increase the anticoagulant (blood-thinning) effects of acenocoumarol, a oral anticoagulant similar to *Warfarin*, but shorter acting—so the effects with ALC will likely be similar.[8,9] This interaction has only been reported with L-carnitine, but theoretically could occur with ALC supplementation.

DOSAGE

Research has shown that diabetics who take 1,000 milligrams of ALC a day show the best response from supplementation.

Alpha Lipoic Acid

Alpha lipoic acid (ALA) is a natural antioxidant produced by the body. It is similar to some vitamins, such as thiamine. Unlike most other antioxidants, however, ALA has the advantage of being soluble in both fat and water, so it can provide protection in the body both inside and outside of cells.[10] ALA is also found in some foods, particularly liver and yeast.

According to studies, taking 600 to 1,200 milligrams oral or intravenous of ALA daily reduced symptoms of peripheral neuropathy in diabetics.[11,12] Additionally, studies showed that ALA improved many of the symptoms associated with DNs, such as burning, pain, numbness, and prickling of the feet and legs.[13,14] ALA also seems to improve objective measures, such as ratings of nerve function decline and disability.[15,16] Among patients, symptom improvement was generally reported within three to five weeks of beginning oral or intravenous dosing.[17-19] Furthermore, other research shows that ALA can contribute to lowering blood sugar levels and insulin sensitivity.[20-23] Theoretically, use with other hypoglycemic drugs might cause additive blood sugar-lowering effects.[24]

DOSAGE

A daily dosage of 600 to 1,200 milligrams of ALA is likely to yield positive results. Doses lower than 600 milligrams daily have not been shown to be effective.[25] However, skin rash has been reported in some individuals after using oral doses of ALA.[26]

Benfotiamin

Benfotiamin is a particularly well-absorbed form of vitamin B_1. Double-blind research in diabetics over a period of three weeks revealed that oral doses of 400 milligrams a day resulted in a statistically significant improvement in neuropathy score in the treatment group when compared to those who took a placebo. The score included both the physician's and the patient's own assessment, and examined various symptoms associated with neuropathy. The most significant improvement reported was pain decrease in polyneuropathy (a type of peripheral neuropathy).[27]

Other research has demonstrated statistically significant effectiveness in reducing diabetic neuropathy pain with daily doses ranging between 150 and 320 milligrams of benfotiamine.[28] In addition, studies have also shown that benfotiamine, when combined with other B vitamins, is effective in the treatment of DNs.[29]

DOSAGE

Benfotiamin has a good tolerance profile without any adverse effects, and there are no established drug interactions associated with this supplement. The best results will likely be seen with 400 milligrams of benfotiamin a day.

Gamma Linolenic Acid

Gamma linolenic acid (GLA) is an omega-6 fatty acid commonly found in evening primrose oil (which is derived from the seeds of the evening primrose plant), as well as in black currant seed oil and borage oil. After consuming GLA, the body converts it into an anti-inflammatory, hormone-like substance called "prostaglandin E1," which is very beneficial to diabetics with DNs.

Results from double-blind research on GLA showed that taking oral doses of 360 to 480 milligrams of GLA daily for six months to one year reduced symptoms and prevented nerve deterioration in peripheral neuropathy patients who had type-1 or type-2 diabetes.[30-33] However, supplementation seems to be more effective in patients with adequate glucose control compared to patients with poor glucose control.[34]

When taken orally, GLA can cause mild gastrointestinal effects such as nausea, vomiting, soft stools, diarrhea, flatulence, and belching.[35-37] Since it has mild blood-thinning properties, GLA might prolong bleeding time if you happen to be injured. Additionally, taking GLA with other anticoagulant or antiplatelet drugs may increase the risk of bruising and bleeding if you happened to be injured.[38]

In addition to DNs, GLA has proven to be beneficial in the treatment of eczema, fibrocystic breast disease, premenstrual syndrome, and rheumatoid arthritis.[39-42]

DOSAGE

Diabetics should take 360 to 480 milligrams of GLA daily in order to see optimal results. It may take six months or longer for results to start showing.

Methylcobalamin

Methylcobalamin is a well-absorbed form of vitamin B_{12}. Double-blind research has shown that daily oral supplementation with 1,500 micrograms of methylcobalamin by diabetics resulted in significant improvements in autonomic neuropathy, when compared to those who took a placebo. The improvements were primarily in physical symptoms and involuntary movements, and signs of regression in diabetic neuropathy were seen.[43] Other research also demonstrated similar benefits and improvements in autonomic neuropathy when methyl-cobalamin was given orally or as an injection.[44,45]

Orally and intramuscularly (an injection into the muscle), vitamin B_{12} or methylcobalamin does not usually cause adverse effects, even when taken in large doses. Limited case reports suggest that chloramphenicol (an antimicrobial drug) can delay or interrupt the response of immature red blood cells to supplemental vitamin B_{12} in some patients.[46]

DOSAGE

A daily dose of 1,500 micrograms of methylcobalamin is appropriate.

You can use any or all of the dietary supplements indicated in this section at the same time. Other than the adverse reactions listed, there are none associated with the concurrent use of more than one supplement.

COMPLEMENTARY TREATMENTS

Complementary and alternative medicine (CAM) therapies have become increasingly popular among people with chronic nerve disorders, including those with DNs. In a study conducted on 180 people who had peripheral neuropathy, 43 percent reported using CAMs.[47] According to the study, the CAM therapies most frequently used were dietary supplements, magnets, acupuncture, herbal remedies, and chiropractic manipulation. About 48 percent of the patients who participated in the study tried more than one form of alternative treatment. Among the patients using CAM therapies, 27 percent felt that their neuropathy symptoms improved with these approaches.

Results from the study also showed that the patients who used CAM were slightly younger than the ones who didn't.

More often than not, the CAM users were college educated. Patients with DN used CAM more frequently than others. Those with burning nerve pain were also more likely to try CAM. Finally, almost half of the patients did *not* consult a physician before starting CAM.

Please don't make the same mistake. If you are considering using CAM therapies, please make sure your healthcare provider is aware of what you are doing. You can even bring this book with you during an office visit to show your healthcare provider what you have in mind.

In this section, you will learn about some complementary treatment options that have been proven to be effective in the treatment of DNs. However, you should still consult your healthcare provider before you begin any of these therapies.

If you would like a more detailed description of any of the therapies discussed in this section, see Appendix C on page 175.

Acupoint Massage

Acupoint massage is a form of massaging that is based on the principles of acupuncture. In a twelve-week study of eighty-two patients with diabetic peripheral neuropathy (DPN), the effects of a medicated bath plus an acupoint massage on limbs were investigated for effectiveness.[48] The type of medication used was not indicated. The test subjects were divided into two groups—both received conventional Western medical treatment for DPN, but one of the groups also received the acupoint massage. The results showed that the people who received the acupoint massage in addition to medication had a much higher rate of effectiveness in treating their DPN (81 percent improvement, compared to a 52.5 percent improvement). Additionally, nerve transmission speed (the speed at which one nerve cell communicates information to another) improved more for those in the acupoint massage group.

Acupuncture

Acupuncture is an ancient Chinese therapy that involves inserting needles into specific points in the body in order to relieve pain.[49] A number of studies have been done showing that acupuncture can be effective in the treatment of DPN. In one study, ninety patients with DPN received wrist-ankle acupuncture, whole body acupuncture, or conventional medical treatment with pain medication.[50] The two acupuncture groups experienced significantly better results than the conventional medical group. This included improvements in the metabolism of blood glucose and blood lipids, lowering blood viscosity, and restoring the functions of peripheral nerve cells.

In another study, forty-four patients with DPN received six courses of acupuncture for a ten-week period.[51] The results were that 77 percent of the patients experienced significant symptom improvement, and 15 percent reported a complete elimination of symptoms. At the beginning of the study, 63 percent of the patients were using standard medications. During the follow-up period after the study, 67 percent of those patients reported they had been able to decrease or discontinue their medications.

In a series of sixty-eight case studies (involving a total of sixty-eight DPN patients treated with acupuncture), forty-three of the patients experienced marked improvement, twenty experienced some improvement, and only five exhibited no improvement.[52]

Also, a study compared two styles of acupuncture—the traditional Chinese medicine and Japanese acupuncture—for the treatment of painful diabetic neuropathy.[53] The results showed that both methods lowered pain.

Exercise

If you are suffering from DN, the idea of exercising may not seem all that appealing to you, since you are dealing with pain. This is understandable. Nevertheless, exercise has significant value for people with DN, and if you are able to work out a regime that fits your needs, you will see—and feel—positive results.

Exercise helps increase circulation and stimulates the growth of new vessels, which slow the progression of the neuropathy. It also helps to increase your pain threshold while providing a distraction from nerve pain in your feet. In addition, exercise helps control blood sugar, which can slow down the neuropathy-related nerve damage. Furthermore, exercise can increase insulin sensitivity and insulin levels in type-2 diabetics.[54]

However, with the burning, tingling, and numbness in the extremities (especially the feet) that accompany DN, exercise can be painful. In addition to foot problems, blood pressure problems, or other problems associated with DN, may people have concerns about exercising safely. So, what is the answer to this conundrum? People with DNs can exercise—but they should certainly see their healthcare provider beforehand.

The visit to your healthcare provider should include a thorough exam of your feet, which will help determine which exercises are and are not appropriate for you to do. For example, your healthcare provider may decide that you need to avoid repetitive, weight-bearing exercises since repetitive stress on DN feet may lead to ulcers, fractures, and joint deformities.[55] In this case, you may be instructed to avoid jogging, prolonged walking, and step aerobics. For these types of DN sufferers, alternative exercises that don't put excessive stress on the feet may be preferred, such as swimming, bicycling, rowing, seated exercises, arm and upper-body exercises, and other non-weight-bearing exercises.

It is important to know that each person's exercise program should be personalized for his or her needs. Some people use self-monitored walking programs as an exercise of choice. In one twelve-month, randomized, controlled study, a self-monitored walking program combined with diabetic foot care education and regular foot care did not lead to significant increases in foot ulcers in DN patients. Those participating in the walking program also performed leg strengthening and balance exercises, and received motivational telephone calls every two weeks.[56] An example of a successful walking program is the case where a sixty-two-year-old obese diabetic man who had neuropathy, retinopathy, kidney problems, circulation problems, and high blood fats was treated using a combination of medication, diet, and simple walking. As a result, his DN and circulation improved.[57] Furthermore, research has shown that type-2 diabetics can increase insulin sensitivity and insulin levels from exercising more often, without necessarily increasing the intensity or duration of their workouts.[58]

Of course, that is not to say that people with DN won't benefit from a program that includes some level of intense exercise. In one study, type-2 diabetic patients with DN participated in a combined resistance and interval exercise training program (interval training involves mixing high intensity bursts of exercise with moderate intensity recovery periods). The results showed that muscle strength and workload capacity increased, while blood pressure and blood sugar decreased.[59] However, this type of program is not for all people with DN. It is important to be evaluated before starting an exercise program so you will become aware of what exercise your body can handle.

Even when DN patients have a specific foot problem, it is still possible to design an exercise program to fit his or her limitations. For example, many people with DN require extra protection of the forefoot. One study found that biking and stair climbing offer optimal pressure reductions for these types of people. On the contrary, recumbent biking, stair climbing, and elliptical training provide greater protection for the heel.[60] No matter what your needs, your healthcare provider should be able to help you identify an exercise program that will be safe and effective for your individual needs.

Magnet Therapy

Magnet therapy is a complementary and alternative medicine practice involving the use of magnetic fields or electromagnetic radiation. In one study, pulsed magnetic field therapy was used to treat twenty-four subjects with peripheral neuropathy (PN) of various types, including DPN. In the study, the most symptomatic foot in each subject received treatment, while the other foot served as a control.[61] After nine one-hour treatments for nine days (weekends off), the results showed that average pain decreased in the treated foot by 21 percent. After a thirty-day follow-up, patients reported a 49 percent decrease—despite the fact that treatment had been discontinued thirty days prior.

Additionally, in a 4-month, multi-center, double-blind, placebo-controlled study, 375 patients with DPN wore either magnetic insoles or placebo (non-magnetized) insoles in their shoes continuously for the duration of the study.[62] The results showed significant decreases in feelings of burning, numbness, and tingling of the feet in months three and four of the study for those who wore the magnetized insoles.

Moxibustion

Moxibustion is a therapy in which a moxa stick is held 2 to 3 centimeters (cm) above a selected point on the skin until the skin is red. In a study on sixty patients with DPN, the effects of mild-warm (as opposed to hot) moxibustion, acupuncture, and medication were compared as treatment strategies.[63] Patients were divided into three groups of twenty each. The same acupoints (locations on the body) were used in the mild-warm moxibustion group and the acupuncture group. The medication group was treated with Mecobalamin tablets, a coenzyme form of vitamin B_{12}. The results showed a 90 percent improvement in the mild-warm moxibustion group, similar results in the acupuncture group, and much less improvement in the medication group.

Yoga

Yoga is a combination of breathing exercises, physical postures, and meditation aimed at training the consciousness to promote control of the body and mind. In one study, forty subjects with mild-to-moderate DN were treated with either thirty to forty minutes of yoga or light exercise (such as walking) daily for forty days.[64] Improvements were assessed by examining nerve conduction velocity (NCV), a common measurement used to evaluate the function of sensory nerves with regard to numbness, tingling, and burning sensations, both before and after the forty day study. The results showed slight improvements in NCV for both right and left hands in the yoga group, while NCV in the light exercise group continued to deteriorate.

As with dietary supplements, you may also try more than one complementary medicine treatment at the same time. Just be careful not to overextend yourself. If you are experiencing too much pain or discomfort, slow down and reassess the situation.

CONCLUSION

At one time, nerve damage, like the type diabetics with DN experience, was thought to be permanent, with no hope of repair. However, we now know that neuroregeneration in the peripheral nervous system (the hands and feet) actually occurs to a significant degree with treatment.[65] Therefore, taking measures to reduce the decline of nerve function and stimulating the growth of new vessels to help slow the progression of the neuropathy (as in the case of exercising), may help not only with DN symptoms, but may also have the potential to help support long-term healthy nerve function.

In other words, you don't have to accept DN and its pain as a permanent reality in your life. There are things you can do to alleviate your pain and discomfort, minimizing suffering and making life more enjoyable.

CHAPTER 6

CARDIOVASCULAR ISSUES

Most diabetics have an increased risk for heart disease and stroke, due to high blood pressure, cholesterol, and triglyceride levels—associated with complications from diabetes—which can all result in death. In fact, more than 65 percent of people with diabetes die from heart disease or stroke—quite a grim statistic. The good news is, however, that by managing diabetes, high blood pressure, and blood lipids (cholesterol and triglycerides), diabetics can greatly reduce these cardiovascular risks.[1]

In this chapter, the importance of diet when dealing with diabetes (which was discussed in Chapter 2) will be re-examined, with a focus on reducing cardiovascular risk. Next, we will take a look at specific dietary supplements that may help control blood pressure, cholesterol, and triglyceride levels. Finally, complementary treatments that have also been shown to be beneficial for these cardiovascular issues will also be discussed.

DIET AND CARDIOVASCULAR DISEASE

Although Chapter 2 addresses the significance of diet for diabetics, I would be remiss if I did not briefly recount the incredibly important role diet plays in cardiovascular health. Specifically, the issues of high blood pressure, high cholesterol, and high triglycerides—all complications of diabetes—can be largely and successfully addressed by adopting a diet plan.

In this section, you will be introduced to the best dietary option that works for these purposes: the Mediterranean diet.

The Mediterranean Diet

The Mediterranean diet is based upon the diets of at least sixteen countries that border the Mediterranean Sea. Although there are many differences in culture, ethnic background, religion, economy, and agricultural production that result in variations in food intake among the population groups, there is still a common Mediterranean dietary pattern that includes the following guidelines:

• Dairy products, fish, and poultry are consumed in low-to-moderate amounts

• Eggs are consumed zero to four times a week

• High consumption of fruits, vegetables, bread and other cereals, potatoes, beans, nuts, and seeds

• Little red meat is eaten

• Olive oil is an important monounsaturated fat source

• Wine is consumed in low-to-moderate amounts

Although the Atkins, Zone, Sugar Busters!, and South Beach diets have data proving that they are effective for weight loss (at least for the short-term) and do not generally increase harmful disease-oriented outcomes, they have little evidence of patient-oriented benefits. On the contrary, there is extensive patient-oriented outcome data that show the Mediterranean diet plays a significant role in risk reduction and mortality rates of fatal and nonfatal heart attacks.[2] Strong evidence supports Mediterranean dietary patterns, including intake of vegetables and nuts, as protective against coronary heart disease.[3]

In addition, there is strong evidence for the protective effect of monounsaturated fatty acids and prudent dietary patterns.[4] A prudent diet consists of lots of vegetables, fruits, beans, whole grains, and fish. Research clearly demonstrates that the people who follow this diet are at low risk for cardiovascular disease.

The people at high risk for cardiovascular disease are those who eat the typical Western diet, which is loaded with red meat, processed meat, refined grains, sweets, desserts, fried foods, and high-fat dairy products.[5,6] Furthermore, strong evidence has also shown a clear, harmful relationship between cardiovascular disease and the intake of trans-fatty acids and foods with a high glycemic index or load.[7]

In 2006, the American Heart Association released guidelines integrating recommendations from a variety of diets into a single plan. The guidelines stated the emphasis should be on diets rich in fruits, vegetables, and healthful fatty acids. Additionally, the ideal diet should limit saturated fat intake. A stepwise individualized approach may be a practical way to help reduce your cardiovascular disease risk.[8,9]

DIETARY SUPPLEMENTS

There are a number of dietary supplements that can help manage high blood pressure and blood lipids. Specifically, artichoke leaf extract, beta-sitosterol, coenzyme Q-10, green tea extract, pantethine, and sitostanol show particular promise in these areas.

Artichoke Leaf Extract

Not to be confused with the culinary treat of steamed or grilled artichokes dipped in butter, the herbal extract version of artichoke leaf (sans the butter) has medicinal properties. Aside from its well-established effects for promoting liver health and its popular use in Europe for treating mild indigestion, artichoke leaf extract also has the ability to reduce total and LDL ("bad" cholesterol) cholesterol, and the LDL/HDL (HDL is considered "good" cholesterol) ratio over a six to twelve-week period.

In one double-blind, placebo-controlled study, 143 adult patients with initial total cholesterol of at least 280 mg/dL were given either artichoke leaf extract or a placebo. Those using artichoke leaf extract experienced an 18.5 percent decrease in total cholesterol, compared to the 8.6 percent decrease experienced by the placebo group. The LDL-cholesterol decreased levels 22.9 percent in the artichoke group and 6.3 percent for the placebo group, and the LDL/HDL ratio (the ratio of bad-to-good cholesterol) showed a decrease of 20.2 percent in the artichoke group and 7.2 percent in the placebo group—a very positive result.[10] Other research has shown similar results, some even stating that artichoke left extract may have an even greater effect in people with higher cholesterol levels.[11]

DOSAGE

The typical dose used in research is between 1,800 and 1,920 milligrams per day taken in two to three divided doses. When taken orally, artichoke extract might increase flatulence in some patients.

Beta-Sitosterol

Beta-sitosterol is a plant sterol. Plant sterols are natural substances found in small quantities in many fruits, vegetables, nuts, seeds, cereals, legumes, vegetable oils, and other plant sources. Research has demonstrated that taking beta-sitosterol orally significantly reduces total and LDL cholesterol levels, but has little or no effect on HDL cholesterol.

Beta-sitosterol works by blocking cholesterol absorption in the intestines, which results in lowered LDL cholesterol in the bloodstream. For the most part, consuming about 2 grams a day has been reported to decrease LDL cholesterol by 9 to 20 percent, although doses have ranged between 800 milligrams to 6 grams per day. Doses are given before meals.

Beta-sitosterol is typically given in conjunction with a low-fat diet.[12–21] Orally, beta-sitosterol is usually well tolerated. *Ezetimibe* (Zetia), a medication used to lower cholesterol levels, inhibits intestinal absorption of beta-sitosterol.

DOSAGE

For most people, 800 to 2,000 milligrams of beta-sitosterol per day, in divided doses taken before meals, is a good amount.

Coenzyme Q-10

Although structurally related to vitamin K, coenzyme Q-10 (CoQ10) is not a vitamin, but rather a coenzyme that helps to utilize oxygen as part of its important role in cellular energy metabolism. Research has also shown that CoQ10 functions in a number of other beneficial ways, including free radical scavenging.[22] In double-blind research, supplementation with 200 milligrams of CoQ10 daily significantly lowered systolic and diastolic blood pressure by several points, and also improved long-term blood glucose control in subjects with type-2 diabetes. (During each heartbeat, blood pressure varies between a maximum, or systolic—the number on top of a blood pressure reading—and a minimum, or diastolic—the number on the bottom of a blood pressure reading).[23] In other double-blind research, hypertension patients with insulin resistance—who were currently using antihypertensive medication—experienced significantly lower blood pressure (by several points) with 120 milligrams of CoQ10. These patients also experienced reductions in insulin resistance, glucose levels, triglyceride levels, and lipid peroxides.[24] Other research has shown similar results.[25] CoQ10 is generally well tolerated, and may have additive blood pressure-lowering effects when used with antihypertensive drugs.

DOSAGE

An optimum dose of CoQ10 is 200 milligrams daily, although benefits have been seen from taking as little as 30 milligrams a day.

Green Tea Extract

Although green tea is made from the leaves of the same plant that brings us ordinary black tea, green tea is less fermented and therefore contains far more polyphenol catechins and theaflavins, natural ingredients that give green tea its medicinal properties. Green tea extract is more concentrated than a cup of green tea, but both essentially have the same medicinal properties.

In double-blind research, seventy-eight obese women received either green tea extract or a placebo for twelve weeks. The results were that the green tea extract group had a significant reduction in LDL-cholesterol and triglycerides, and marked increase in the level of HDL-cholesterol (the "good cholesterol"). On the other hand, the placebo group showed significant reduction in triglycerides only. In one study, the group of people taking green tea extract (1,200 milligrams a day) had significant reduction in LDL cholesterol and triglycerides, while also experiencing marked increase in HDL cholesterol.[26] In another study, participants were given 583 milligrams of catechins (from green tea) a day. These participants experienced a 10 percent decrease in systolic blood pressure and a 9 percent reduction in LDL cholesterol, compared to no change in systolic blood pressure and a 1 percent increase in LDL cholesterol in the control group.[27] Likewise, another study showed that supplementation with 375 milligrans of a theaflavin-enriched green tea extract per day resulted in an 11.3 percent reduction in total cholesterol, a 16.4 percent reduction in LDL cholesterol, and a 2.3 percent increase in HDL cholesterol, while cholesterol levels did not change significantly in the placebo group.[28] Epidemiological research (research on the health of populations) also indicates that adults who consume six or more cups per day of green tea have a 33 percent lower risk of developing type-2 diabetes, compared to those who consume one cup per day or less.[29]

High doses of green tea extract may cause gastrointestinal upset (cramping) and/or central nervous system stimulation (the nervous "jitters") in some people. Theoretically, the caffeine in green tea might contribute central nervous system effects (hyperactivity, restlessness, etc.) with amphetamines, although GTE only provides about 10 to 30 milligrams of caffeine (compared to 100 milligrams in a cup of moderately brewed coffee).

The catechins and caffeine in green tea are reported to have antiplatelet activity, which means, theoretically, green tea might increase the risk of bleeding when used with antiplatelet or anticoagulant drugs.

DOSAGE

The doses used in research ranged between 375 and 1,200 milligrams of green tea extract. Consuming 375 milligrams of green tea extract (providing 60 percent or more polyphenols, which would be indicated on the label of the product) would be equivalent to drinking about six to eight cups of green tea.

Pantethine

Pantethine is a form of pantothenic acid, also know as vitamin B_5. Results from a double-blind study showed taking 900 milligrams of pantethine in three divided doses (300 milligrams three times a day) daily can reduce triglycerides by 30 percent, reduce LDL cholesterol by 13.5 percent, and raise HDL cholesterol by 10 percent in patients with high cholesterol and triglyceride levels.[30] Three other double-blind studies showed similar results.[31-33] In addition, several open studies have specifically examined the use of 600 to 1,200 milligrams of pantethine daily to improve cholesterol and triglyceride levels in diabetics and found it to be safe and effective.[34-36] In one of those studies, 900 milligrams of pantethine daily resulted in a 16 percent reduction in total cholesterol, a 30 percent reduction in very-low-density lipoprotein (VLDL) cholesterol (a very bad from of cholesterol), and a 45 percent reduction in triglycerides after supplementing for two months.[37]

Pantethine seems to be well-tolerated. It may cause minor gastrointestinal complaints in some people such as nausea, diarrhea, and upper abdominal discomfort. Some evidence suggests that pantethine reduces platelet aggregation. When taken concurrently with drugs that affect platelets or coagulation, it might have an additive effect, increasing the risk of bleeding if injured.

DOSAGE

In research, the most frequently used daily dosage is 900 milligrams, taken in divided doses.

Sitostanol

Similar to plant sterols, plant stanols are natural substances that occur in even smaller quantities in many of the same sources as plant sterols. Like sterols, stanols block the absorption of cholesterol in the intestines. One stanol, sitostanol, has been extensively researched for its effect on cholesterol. The results showed that taking sitostanol orally is effective for reducing total and LDL cholesterol in about 88 percent of adult patients when used alone or in combination with a low-fat diet or statin drug (a drug that inhibits the production of cholesterol in the body).[38–53] When used alone, sitostanol can reduce total and LDL cholesterol levels by 10 to 15 percent. When added to statin drugs, sitostanol reduces total cholesterol by 3 to 11 percent and LDL cholesterol by 7 to 16 percent.

Clinical studies have used between 800 milligrams and 4 grams per day for research purposes.[54] Results have shown that the best cholesterol-lowering effects occur with about 2 grams per day. Doses above 2 grams per day do not seem to provide additional benefit.[55] Sitostanols are not currently found in dietary supplements, but they can be found in certain margarine-type spreads and salad dressings. Read product labels in your supermarket and see which of these products provide sitostanol.

Orally, sitostanol seems to be very well-tolerated. It can reduce absorption and blood levels of beta-carotene, so if you are taking beta-carotene supplements, you should take sitostanol at a different time of the day.

DOSAGE

For best results, use 2,000 milligrams of sitostanol in divided doses, taken before meals.

COMPLEMENTARY TREATMENTS

Many of the time-honored approaches in this section have been used for hundreds of years in different cultures to improve cardiovascular health. It is only in recent times that researchers have studied these methods and have documented their effectiveness in scientific research.

In this section, you will learn about a few complementary therapies that have been proven to be successful in lowering the risk of cardiovascular issues in diabetics. Acupuncture (as well as moxibustion and electroacupuncture) has been shown to help lower cholesterol and triglycerides. The effectiveness of Transcendental Meditation (TM), a relatively new therapy that was introduced in 1958, has been validated in over 600 scientific studies, including ones that demonstrate TM's effectiveness in lowering blood pressure. In addition, yoga is a therapy intended to relax the body and help lower blood pressure, cholesterol, and triglycerides.

Of course, exercise is widely accepted as a method for helping to promote a healthy cardiovascular system. Be sure to speak with a healthcare practitioner to determine an appropriate and healthy exercise level for you.

Acupuncture

Acupuncture is a therapy that involves a licensed acupuncturist inserting needles into strategic areas throughout the body. it is believed to help deal with pain, but can have other benefits as well. In an acupuncture study of fifty-four diabetics, patients were randomly divided into an acupuncture group and a control group. For thirty days, the patients in the two groups were all treated with conventional diabetic drug therapy, while those in the acupuncture group also received acupuncture treatment. After the study's conclusion, total cholesterol and triglyceride levels significantly decreased and HDL cholesterol significantly increased in the acupuncture group, when compared to the control group.[56]

Another study compared the effectiveness of acupuncture, moxibustion (see page 178 for a definition), or acupuncture plus moxibustion on seventy-nine type-2 diabetic subjects. After treatment, the clinical symptoms for all three groups significantly improved. Fasting blood glucose, twenty-four-hour urinal glucose, glycosylated hemoglobin, cholesterol, triglyceride, and LDL cholesterol all decreased in varying degrees, while HDL cholesterol increased in all of the three groups. The best effects, however, were seen in the acupuncture plus moxibustion group.[57]

Electroacupuncture (EA) is a form of acupuncture in which the needles are attached to an electric device that generates pulses. In an EA study, fifty-five obese women were divided into three groups: a control group, an EA group, and a diet restriction group. For twenty days, EA was performed on the members in the EA group once daily for thirty minutes (the patients in this group didn't change their diets or anything else). Patients in the diet restriction group followed a 1,425-calorie daily diet plan. The results showed that EA patients experienced a 4.8 percent weight reduction, whereas patients on diet restriction had a 2.5 percent weight reduction. There were significant decreases in total cholesterol and triglyceride levels in both the EA and diet groups when compared to the control group. Finally, there was a greater decrease in LDL cholesterol in the EA group than in the control group.[58]

Exercise

Physical inactivity is a well-established risk factor for cardiovascular disease. Conversely, being physically active can help lower your risk for cardiovascular disease, but most Americans are not physically active enough to gain any health benefits.[59] Swimming, bicycling, jogging, skiing, aerobic dancing, walking, and many other activities can help your heart. Whether it is included in a structured exercise program or as part of your daily routine, physical activity adds up to a healthier heart.

According to the latest joint American Heart Association/ American College of Sports Medicine guidelines on physical activity, all healthy adults between the ages of eighteen and sixty-five should be getting at least thirty minutes of moderate-intensity aerobic activity five days of the week.[60]

Exercise can do much to reduce the risk and help manage various types of cardiovascular disease, such as high blood pressure, coronary heart disease, stroke, and HDL cholesterol modification.[61-64]

Transcendental Meditation (TM)

Transcendental Meditation (TM) is a form of meditation designed to be practiced for twenty minutes twice a day while sitting comfortable with the eyes closed.[65] (For a more detailed definition, see page 180.)

Stress is known to contribute to hypertension, cardiovascular disease, and even death (usually as a result of cardiovascular disease). In a review of the published literature on studies about stress reduction and blood pressure, 17 trials were examined with 960 participants who had hypertension. Different methods of stress reduction were found to have varying degrees of effectiveness in lowering blood pressure. The method with greatest effectiveness and statistical significance was TM, which lowered blood pressure by an average of five points.[66]

Randomized controlled trials, meta-analyses, and other controlled studies indicate that this meditation technique reduces risk factors and can slow or reverse the progression of negative changes underlying cardiovascular disease. Studies with this technique have revealed reductions in blood pressure, artery thickening, heart blockages, mortality, and other relevant outcomes. These effects compare favorably with those of conventional therapy for cardiovascular disease prevention.[67]

Yoga

Yoga is a combination of breathing exercises, physical postures, and meditation aimed at training the consciousness to promote control of the body and mind. Researchers examined sixty-five studies on a variety of meditation practices for common conditions, including hypertension and cardiovascular diseases. The results showed that while various other relaxation techniques significantly reduced blood pressure, yoga helped reduce stress.[68] Since stress is a big risk factor for cardiovascular issues, keeping it to a minimum is wise.

Other studies have found more profound benefits associated with yoga. In a three-month, randomized study, fifty patients with metabolic syndrome (prediabetes) were treated with conventional therapy alone, while another fifty underwent daily yoga and meditation exercises in addition to conventional therapy.[69] The results showed that the yoga/meditation group experienced a significant change in cardiovascular parameters when compared to the conventional therapy-only group. These changes included, on average, a fifty-six-point reduction in fasting blood glucose, a sixteen-point reduction in systolic blood pressure, an eight-point reduction in diastolic blood pressure, a fifty-eight-point decrease in triglycerides, a fifty-one-point decrease in total cholesterol, and a seven-point increase in HDL cholesterol. Similar results were seen in a ten-day study of ninety-eight subjects with hypertension, coronary artery disease, diabetes mellitus, and a variety of other illnesses. These subjects practiced yoga postures, breathing exercises, relaxation techniques, group support, individualized advice, lectures and films on the philosophy of yoga and the place of yoga in daily life, meditation, stress management, nutrition, and knowledge about the illness. The results were that the subjects experienced improvements in blood glucose, total cholesterol, LDL-cholesterol, VLDL-cholesterol, the ratio of total cholesterol to HDL-cholesterol, triglycerides, and HDL-cholesterol.[70]

CONCLUSION

If there is anything you should take away from this chapter, it should be that even if you are diabetic, you have the power to avoid becoming a cardiovascular disease statistic. Even though statistics about Americans and cardiovascular diseases may seem dismal, you should have learned in this chapter that as a group, cardiovascular issues are highly responsive to lifestyle changes. By managing your diabetes, blood pressure, cholesterol, and triglyceride levels, you can keep your risk for cardiovascular complications to a minimum.[71] The information in this chapter is filled with scientifically-proven, effective strategies for doing just that.

CHAPTER 7

CIRCULATION PROBLEMS

When circulation is healthy, blood flows through blood vessels at a good pace. That means blood leaves the heart, travels through arteries, and delivers oxygen and important nutrients to cells via capillaries (the smallest blood vessels). Then, blood is returned to the heart through a network of veins. However, sometimes there are problems that slow circulation down, which can occur when blood vessels are made stiff by plaque, "sludgy" blood (platelets clumping together), and other issues.

Unfortunately, circulation problems are very common in diabetics. Although it is possible for such problems to occur anyplace in the body, the reality of the situation is that they tend to occur almost exclusively in the legs and feet. The reason for this is that the legs and feet are the areas farthest away from the heart, so blood has the farthest distance to circulate in order to reach these sites and return back to the heart. Peripheral vascular disease (PVD) is the medical name given to a group of problems with poor circulation to the feet and legs. Diabetes is one of the main risk factors for PVD. In fact, PVD is twice as common in patients with diabetes than in patients without diabetes. Approximately 20 percent of diabetics will, at some point, develop either a foot infection or ulcer, or will suffer foot pain even though they are at rest. Both of these issues require hospitalization for evaluation and treatment.[1]

PVD is also an important contributory factor in non-healing foot ulcers and amputation in diabetes.[2]

A related circulation problem is intermittent claudication (IC). IC is basically pain or cramps in the leg muscles that occur while walking. They usually go away completely after a few minutes of rest. IC is the first recognizable symptom of PVD. Pain is most commonly felt in the calf, but can occur in the buttocks, thigh, or foot. The next time the same amount of walking or other exercise takes place, the pain will occur again. IC is the most common symptom of PVD, but around two thirds of PVD patients experience no symptoms.[3] This can be problematic, since a lack of symptoms likely means that no additional measures will be taken to care for this disorder. The most severe consequence of lack of care is foot amputation—although before circulation gets that bad there will be some symptoms.

In this chapter, we will first take a look at specific dietary supplements that may help in the treatment of circulatory problems. After that, we will consider other complementary treatments that have also been shown to be beneficial for PVD and/or IC.

DIETARY SUPPLEMENTS

There are a number of dietary supplements that have potential to help in the treatment of PVD and/or IC. Some of the most promising are garlic, Ginkgo biloba extract, inositol nicotinate, L-carnitine or propionyl-L-carnitine, policosanol, and vitamin E. A discussion of each of these supplements, along with the proper dosage, follows.

Garlic

Everyone is familiar with garlic and its pungent aroma. Love it or hate it, garlic has an extensive history of medicinal use in addition to its culinary reputation. One such use is associated with its circulatory and cardiovascular benefits. In particular, a standardized extract of garlic has been tested as a treatment for IC. In one double-blind study on individuals with IC, participants were divided into two groups. One group was given 400 milligrams of a standardized garlic powder extract twice a day for twelve weeks, and the other group was given a placebo. The increase in walking distance was significantly greater in those receiving the standardized garlic powder extract. In fact, they were able to increase their walking distance by about 50 yards (from 176 to 226 yards). That's about 47 percent farther than the placebo group was able to increase their walking distance.[4] In addition, diastolic blood pressure, spontaneous blood clotting, blood plasma thickness, and cholesterol concentration decreased significantly for the participants who supplemented with the garlic extract. An interesting bit of information about the study is that the garlic-specific increase in walking distance did not appear to occur until the fifth week of treatment, simultaneous with the decrease in spontaneous blood clotting. What this means is that garlic may be an especially appropriate agent for the long-term treatment of early IC.

Orally, garlic has dose-related adverse effects, which most commonly include breath and body odor. It might enhance the effects of the blood-thinning medication *Warfarin*, and theoretically might also enhance the effects and adverse effects of other anticoagulant and antiplatelet drugs. It might also decrease the effectiveness of cyclosporine and increase the liver's ability to metabolize certain drugs, including acetaminophen *(Tylenol)*, chlorzoxazone, ethanol, theophylline, and some anesthetics (such as enflurane). Research in animal models suggests that a water extract of garlic can reduce isoniazid (antituberculosis medication) levels by about 65 percent.

Garlic preparations containing the sulfur compound allicin may decrease plasma concentrations of the protease inhibitor saquinavir.

DOSAGE

An effective dose would be 400 milligrams twice daily of standardized garlic extract, providing 2,400 micrograms of allicin (a key sulfur compound in garlic).

Ginkgo Biloba Extract

Ginkgo biloba extract (GBE) is perhaps best known for its beneficial effect on improving short-term memory in age-related memory impairment and dementias (such as Alzheimer's disease). However, the reason that it has this benefit is due to the fact that it improves cerebral circulation. Of interest to diabetics is that GBE also improves peripheral circulation (circulation to the arms and legs).

An analysis was conducted on eight randomized, placebo-controlled, double-blind studies examining the effectiveness of 120 to 160 milligrams of GBE per day for the treatment of IC. The results showed that that GBE was significantly superior to the placebo in treating the symptoms of IC, although the overall treatment effect was modest.[5] Other research has shown that a higher dose of 240 milligrams per day seems to have greater benefit for the treatment of PVD.[6,7]

GBE is well-tolerated in typical doses (10 to 240 milligrams). GBE has been shown to decrease platelet aggregation and might increase the risk of bleeding when combined with antiplatelet or anticoagulant drugs. GBE might decrease the effectiveness of alprazolam *(Xanax)* in some people. Theoretically, in type-2 diabetics, GBE may increase the rate at which the liver metabolizes insulin and other hypoglycemic agents, which can possibly reduce elevated blood glucose. However, in diet-controlled diabetes patients with high insulin levels, GBE did not significantly affect insulin or blood glucose levels.

DOSAGE

A 50:1 Ginkgo biloba extract standardized for 24 percent flavone glycosides and 6 percent terpene lactones should be taken in doses of 120 to 240 milligrams daily. "50:1" means that 50 kilograms of Ginkgo leaves were used to make 1 kilogram of Ginkgo extract. If you are not sure which end of the dosage range to use, start at the lower dose and work your way up if you don't notice benefits at the starting dose.

Inositol Nicotinate

Inositol nicotinate (or inositol hexanicotinate), is a form of the B-vitamin niacin. It gained notoriety due to the fact that it did not cause the severe characteristic "flush" (reddening, warming, and itching of the skin—particularly face, arms, and chest—for about fifteen to twenty minutes) commonly associated with niacin use.

Nevertheless, inositol nicotinate has some of the same circulation-enhancing properties as niacin. This was demonstrated in a placebo-controlled study, where twenty-three patients with Raynaud's disease (a blood vessel disorder affecting blood flow tp the extremities) were given either 4 grams of inositol nicotinate or a placebo daily during cold weather.[8] Improvements in circulation were noted in the inositol nicotinate group, who reported feeling subjectively better and had demonstrably shorter and fewer attacks of vasospasm (a condition in which blood vessels spasm) during the trial period.

In another study of thirty patients with Raynaud's phenomenon—which is less severe than Raynaud's disease—blood flow and the skin's microcirculation was significantly improved by inositol nicotinate, demonstrating effectiveness for improving symptoms of PVD. This study suggests that the therapeutic effect of this drug is not merely due to vasodilation (the expansion of blood vessels), but also to additional mechanisms such as the reduction of fibrin clots and the lowering of blood fat lipids.

Orally, inositol nicotinate was found to be effective, and it was absent of unwanted side effects.[9] Similar research suggests that long-term treatment with inositol nicotinate may result in improvement in peripheral circulation.[10] Several weeks of treatment may be necessary before the full beneficial effects are seen.

Theoretically, concurrent use with anticoagulant and/or antiplatelet drugs might increase the risk of bleeding if injured, due to the fibrinolytic effects of inositol nicotinate. Also, concurrent use with antidiabetic drugs might interfere with blood glucose control.

DOSAGE

The optimal dose for inositol nicotinate is 4,000 milligrams daily, in divided doses (2,000 milligrams twice a day).

L-carnitine or Propionyl-L-carnitine

L-carnitine is an amino acid that is involved in the transport of fatty acids throughout the body. It has demonstrated benefits in cardiovascular research, and, to some extent, in weight loss research. In a double-blind study, 4 grams of L-carnitine daily were given to twenty patients with PVD. The results showed that L-carnitine improved walking distances in people with PVD.[11] In several studies, oral or intravenous administration of propionyl-L-carnitine (a form of L-carnitine) was effective in helping patients with IC and PVD.[12-17] For patients with PVD and IC whose walking distances are restricted to less than 273 yards, propionyl-L-carnitine may increase walking distance and time. Propionyl-L-carnitine does not seem to help milder PVD. Studies used 1,000 milligrams, two or three times daily.[18]

DOSAGE

The dose for L-carnitine is 4,000 milligrams daily, in divided doses (2,000 milligrams twice a day). The dose for propionyl-L-carnitine is 1,000 milligrams, two or three times daily. Start at twice daily, and increase to three times if you don't notice much difference.

Policosanol

Policosanol is a waxy substance that can be derived from sugarcane. Policosanol gained scientific interest when some studies demonstrated it was able to lower cholesterol levels. In addition, policosanol has been shown to benefit circulation as well. In a double-blind study, sixty-two patients with IC received either a placebo or 10 milligrams of policosanol twice a day.[19] The patients' walking distances on a treadmill were assessed before and after six months of treatment. The results showed that both initial distance walked and absolute distance increased significantly for the patients taking policosanol, while both variables remained unchanged in the placebo group.

Another study that used the same dose of policosanol showed similar results.[20] When patients took policosanol continuously for two years, their walking capacity more than doubled. This may be related to policosanol's ability to reduce the stickiness of platelets, which could result in improved circulation.[21,22]

Policosanol is usually well-tolerated. Since it can inhibit platelet aggregation, taking policosanol with other antiplatelet or anticoagulant drugs might increase the risk of bruising and bleeding.

DOSAGE

The correct dose is 10 milligrams of policosanol, twice daily.

Vitamin E

Vitamin E is known both for its antioxidant properties, which protect us against the oxidative damage caused by free radicals, and for its cardiovascular benefits, such as reducing the risk of heart attack. In addition, controlled studies have shown that supplementation with 400 to 600 international units (IU) of vitamin E per day can increase both walking distance and blood flow through the arteries of the lower legs in people with IC.[23,24]

One review article suggested that supplementing with vitamin E for a minimum of four to six months may be necessary before significant improvement is seen.[25]

Vitamin E seldom causes adverse effects. However, concurrent use of vitamin E and anticoagulant or antiplatelet agents might increase the risk of bleeding.

DOSAGE

An appropriate dose of vitamin E is 400 to 600 IU daily, which is considerably higher than the 30 IU daily value.

While garlic, Ginkgo biloba extract, inositol nicotinate, L-carnitine or propionyl-L-carnitine, policosanol, and vitamin E are not the only dietary supplements that have potential for treating PVD or IC, they are the ones that have the most data supporting their use, as well as the least adverse effects or interactions. Certain other supplements that are used for this purpose are sometimes redundant to nutrients found in multivitamins, have no research for oral use (only intravenous), or require such a high dose that you would be popping pills all day long to accommodate, which is why I chose not to feature them in this book.

COMPLEMENTARY TREATMENTS

Many people with PVD and IC have tried, or at least considered, one or more complementary or alternative medicine treatment options. Research has shown that the most popular treatments for this purpose are acupressure, acupuncture, biofeedback, exercise, and carbon dioxide (CO_2) applications. However, CO_2 applications are not commonly available in the United States.[26] The other therapies are far more popularized and have varying degrees of effectiveness. Their role in the treatment of PVD and IC will be reviewed in this section.

Acupressure and Acupuncture

Acupressure is a combination of acupuncture and pressure. In acupressure, physical pressure is applied to acupuncture points on the body instead of inserting needles. In one study, thirty patients with PVD received acupressure, with key acupressure points being stimulated for three minutes.[27] The results were that blood flow to the chest wall, part of the leg, and the upper part of the foot increased significantly during acupressure. Moreover, the blood flow to the lower limbs that had undergone surgery to destroy certain nerves also increased significantly. All in all, acupressure was found to cause significant increases in circulation to the lower limbs in people with PVD.

Acupuncture, which uses needles instead of applying pressure, has also been proven effective for circulatory problems. In a study of fifty-five type-2 diabetic patients with PVD, a course of ten acupuncture sessions were administered.[28] The results were that 78 percent of the diabetics experienced improvements in blood flow and artery circumference (the "openness" of the artery).

Biofeedback

Biofeedback is a technique in which various monitoring devices are used to help a person learn to voluntarily alter body functions that are normally involuntary, such as brain activity, blood pressure, muscle tension, or heart rate. A prospective, randomized study was designed to determine the effects of biofeedback-assisted relaxation training on the healing of foot ulcers (which, as stated, can be caused by the circulatory issues many diabetics face).[29] The study was conducted on thirty-two diabetics, each with a foot ulcer. While those in the control group received only traditional medical care, the experimental group received the same traditional medical care combined with a biofeedback-assisted relaxation training program designed to increase blood circulation to the feet. In the experimental group, fourteen of the sixteen ulcers (87.5 percent) healed, while in the control group, only seven out of sixteen (43.8 percent) healed.

Regarding thermal biofeedback, researchers from the Center for the Study of Complementary and Alternative Therapies at the University of Virginia have stated:

> Thermal biofeedback, however, alone or in conjunction with other mind-body techniques, improves peripheral circulation, pain, neuropathy, ulcer healing, ambulatory activity, and quality of life. It is noninvasive, inexpensive, and consistent with community-based approaches to diabetes self-management. As an adjunct to the medical management of diabetes, thermal biofeedback may help ameliorate some of the vascular complications.[30]

In a case study, the therapeutic effects of thermal biofeedback on a patient with type-2 diabetes, vascular disease, and symptoms of IC were examined.[31] The patient received ther-

mal biofeedback from the hand for five sessions, then from the
foot for sixteen sessions. Hand and foot skin temperatures
were monitored simultaneously. In addition, the patient practiced daily at home. Follow-up measurements were taken after
twelve months, and then again after forty-eight months. The
results were that foot temperature rose specifically in response
to foot temperature biofeedback. Starting foot temperature
rose between sessions. After-treatment blood pressure was
reduced to a normal level. Attacks of IC were reduced to zero
after twelve sessions, and walking distance increased by about
a mile per day over the course of treatment.

Exercise

Supervised exercise is a major treatment for patients with
PVD, and it is a relatively inexpensive, low-risk option compared with other more invasive therapies.[32] In fact, in a
review of 22 studies including 1,200 IC patients, exercise
(specifically, treadmill walking) significantly improved maximum walking time by approximately 50 to 200 percent, and
improved pain-free walking distances when compared to
usual care or a placebo.[33] In these cases, usual care consisted
of surgical intervention, angioplasty, antiplatelet and drug
therapy, or pneumatic foot and calf compression (wraps and
special garments).

It should also be noted that aging affects the function and
structure of arteries and increases the risk of cardiovascular
disease (CVD), which includes PVD. Specifically, large arteries
become stiffer and less elastic. Studies have shown that adults
who regularly perform aerobic exercise (such as walking) tend
to have less or no increases in artery stiffness when compared
to those who don't exercise. In fact, regular aerobic exercise
favorably impacts aging of arteries, which in turn preserves
blood vessel function and may reduce the risk of CVD. These

positive results, while seen with aerobic exercise, are not evident in resistance training, such as weight-lifting.[34]

CONCLUSION

Circulation problems are a prevalent, long-term complication of uncontrolled high blood glucose levels, with one of the most severe possible permanent outcomes—foot amputation. That's the bad news. The good news is that diabetes-related circulation problems can be greatly reduced or eliminated by simply incorporating a little bit of regular exercise and the use of a few dietary supplements (along with sensible dietary modification measures) into your daily routine.

CHAPTER 8

EYE HEALTH AND DIABETES

When it comes to diabetes and eye health, it is important to know that anyone who has type-1 or type-2 diabetes is at risk of developing diabetic retinopathy.

Diabetic retinopathy is the result of damage to the tiny blood vessels of the retina (back of the eye). Poor blood glucose control and an over-accumulation of glucose and/or fructose are the main causes of damage to these blood vessels. The damage makes the retinal blood vessels become more permeable, and less strong.[1] As the disease progresses, a lack of oxygen in the retina causes fragile, new, blood vessels to grow along the retina and in the clear, gel-like vitreous humour that fills the inside of the eye. Without timely treatment, these new blood vessels can bleed, cloud vision, and destroy the retina, which can eventually lead to blindness.

Diabetic retinopathy is a serious complication of diabetes. It is one of the leading causes of new cases of blindness in the adult population worldwide. In type-1 diabetics, almost all patients develop some signs of retinopathy in the first twenty years of having diabetes. In type-2 diabetics, up to 30 percent of patients already have retinopathy at diagnosis, increasing to over 60 percent within the first twenty years. Additionally, diabetics are 25 times more likely to go blind as a result of retinopathy than non-diabetics suffering from the disease are. Therefore, it is very important for diabetics to understand what diabetic retinopathy is and to be aware of its symptoms.

107

In this chapter, we will first examine the symptoms of diabetic retinopathy, because it is very important that all diabetics know what to look for when dealing with this serious complication. Next, we will take a look at specific dietary supplements that may help in the treatment of diabetic retinopathy. Finally, we will consider other complementary treatments that have also been shown to be beneficial for this disorder.

SYMPTOMS OF DIABETIC RETINOPATHY

The most important thing to know about diabetic retinopathy is that during the initial stages of the disease, most people do not notice any change in their vision, nor do they feel any pain. Therefore, do *not* wait for symptoms to show up. If you are a diabetic, you should have a comprehensive dilated eye exam *at least* once a year.

When the first symptom does occur, it will most likely be blurred vision caused by the macula swelling from leaking fluid (otherwise known as macula edema). The macula is the part of the retina that provides sharp central vision.

Other symptoms may occur as a result of new blood vessels growing on the surface of the retina, bleeding into the eye, and blocking vision. Typically, you will first start to see "spots" that seem to float in your vision. These "spots" are actually specks of blood, so if they occur, you should see your eye care professional as soon as possible. You may need treatment before more serious bleeding occurs. In fact, hemorrhages tend to occur more than once, and often during sleep.

Even if the spots clear before you get treatment, you should still see your eye care professional at the first sign of blurred vision, before more bleeding occurs.

The most common treatable risk factors for diabetic retinopathy are hyperglycemia (high blood glucose levels) and hypertension (high blood pressure).[2] In addition, higher plasma total homocysteine concentration (a risk factor in heart disease) was observed more in diabetic individuals with retinopathy than in those without retinopathy, so this may also be a treatable risk factor to consider.[3]

DIETARY SUPPLEMENTS

There are a number of dietary supplements that have potential to help in the treatment of diabetic retinopathy. Some of the most promising are bilberry fruit extract, Ginkgo biloba extract, OPC, folic acid, and vitamin B_{12}. A discussion of each of these follows.

Bilberry Fruit Extract

Bilberry (Vaccinium myrtillus), also known as European blueberry, has been used as a food for centuries. It became widely known to herbalists in the sixteenth century when its use was documented for promoting urinary tract, liver, and respiratory health.

Modern research has focused on bilberry's benefits for supporting eye health, vascular health, and healthy blood glucose levels.[4] Bilberry's naturally occurring active components act as antioxidants in the retina of the eye, making it a potential preventive measure against oxidative damage to the macula and lens of the eye.[5] Bilberry has also been shown to strengthen capillaries in the retina.[6]

A special report on bilberry discussed a double-blind study in which fourteen patients with diabetic and/or hypertensive retinopathy (damage to the retina due to high blood pressure) were supplemented with either 115 milligrams of bilberry extract or a placebo daily for one month.[7,8] Significant improvements were observed in the eye function of eleven of the fourteen subjects who received bilberry, and twelve of the fourteen patients showed improvement in the interior structures of the eye, especially the retina.

In another study, thirty-one patients with various types of retinopathy were investigated to determine the effect of bilberry anthocyanosides on the retinal blood vessels.[9] Especially in patients with diabetic retinopathy, a positive influence on the permeability and tendency to hemorrhage was observed.

Clinical studies of bilberry's effectiveness have used formulations containing 25 percent of the bioflavonoid complex anthocyanoside. No adverse effects have been reported from bilberry use. However, concurrent use of bilberry with anti-diabetes drugs might require dosing adjustment of those drugs since preliminary animal research suggests that bilberry extract might have blood glucose lowering activity (which would be a potentially positive interaction).

DOSAGE

A typical amount used in studies is 240 to 480 milligrams per day of bilberry extract in capsules or tablets standardized to 25 percent anthocyanosides.

Ginkgo Biloba Extract

An extract from the leaf of the Ginkgo biloba tree has been studied extensively with regard to promoting cognitive function and short-term memory. In addition, Ginkgo biloba extract also has benefits for diabetic retinopathy.

In a six-month, double-blind trial, twenty-nine diabetic subjects with early diabetic retinopathy received either 160 milligrams Ginkgo biloba extract (GBE) or a placebo.[10] The results showed statistically significant improvements in measures of color vision in the GBE group, and a worsening of measures in the placebo group.

In a three-month study, twenty-five type-2 diabetic patients with retinopathy received 240 milligrams of GBE daily.[11] The results from this study showed a significant reduction in blood viscosity ("sludgy" blood), viscoelasticity (exhibiting both viscosity and elastic characteristics when undergoing deformation), and oxidative stress of blood cells. Additionally, results also showed an increase in retinal capillary blood flow.

GBE is well tolerated in typical doses (see "Dosage" section below). GBE has been shown to decrease platelet aggregation and might increase the risk of bleeding when combined with antiplatelet or anticoagulant drugs. Additionally, GBE might decrease the effectiveness of alprazolam *(Xanax)* in some people.

For type-2 diabetics, GBE may increase the rate at which the liver metabolizes insulin and other hypoglycemic agents, possibly resulting in reduced elevated blood glucose. However, in diet-controlled diabetics with high insulin levels, taking GBE did not significantly affect insulin or blood glucose levels.

DOSAGE

Ginkgo biloba extract should be taken in doses of 240 milligrams per day. Look for a product where the Ginkgo extract is standardized for 24 percent flavone glycosides and 6 percent terpene lactones.

Oligomeric Proanthocyanidins

Oligomeric Proanthocyanidins (OPCs) are a class of natural polyphenols found naturally in grape seeds or pine bark. They are used in dietary supplements.

In a double-blind study, forty patients with retinopathy caused by diabetes, atherosclerosis, or central venous thrombosis were given either a placebo or 50 milligrams of pycnogenol (the trade name for an OPC extract from the bark of the French maritime pine tree) three times a day for two months.[12] The results showed that the pycnogenol slowed or prevented further deterioration of retinal function in patients, while retinopathy and visual acuity in the placebo group progressively worsened.

Additionally, a special report on OPCs reported a review in which twenty-six case studies revealed that OPCs significantly improved vascular lesions, microaneurisms, and excess eye fluid associated with diabetic retinopathy.[13,14]

Grape seed extract and pycnogenol are well tolerated. Known drug interactions are all based upon the use of grape juice, not grape seed extract. However, pycnogenol may interfere with immunosuppressant therapy because of its immuno-stimulating activity.

DOSAGE

150 milligrams of OPCs from grape seed extract or pycnogenol would be an effective daily dose.

Vitamin B$_{12}$ and Folic Acid

Vitamin B$_{12}$ and folic acid belong to the family of B vitamins and play a role in energy metabolism. In addition, they play a role in cardiovascular health.

In a study of fifty diabetics, blood was drawn to determine the diabetics' vitamin B$_{12}$ and folic acid status. There was a statistically significant decrease of serum vitamin B$_{12}$ and folic acid levels and a significant increase of plasma total homocysteine levels in diabetics who had retinopathy in comparison to those without retinopathy.[15] The authors of the study suggest that the homocysteine increase may have been caused by a deficiency of both of these vitamins, and that physicians should recommend vitamin B$_{12}$ and folic acid as replacement therapy in diabetics to prevent future athero-sclerosis and diabetic complications that may be due to high homocysteine levels.

In a study that was conducted in 1958, 100 micrograms per day of vitamin B$_{12}$ were added to the insulin injections of fifteen children who had diabetic retinopathy.[16] After one year, signs of retinopathy disappeared in seven of fifteen cases; after two years, eight of fifteen were free of retinopathy. Given the previously observed higher plasma total homocysteine concentration in diabetic individuals with retinopathy (compared to those without retinopathy), it has been determined that supplementation with vitamin B_{12} and folic acid to lower homocysteine levels can be beneficial.[17]

Additionally, research indicates that supplementation with folic acid at .5 to 5 milligrams per day lowers fasting homocysteine levels by an average of 25 percent, and adding vitamin B_{12} (mean dose of .5 milligrams per day) produces an additional decrease in homocysteine levels of about 7 percent on average.[18]

Vitamin B_{12} is well-tolerated. There are no known interactions that vitamin B_{12} has upon any drugs. Folic acid is well-tolerated in amounts found in fortified foods and supplements in doses less than 1,000 micrograms per day. There is, however, some evidence that folic acid supplements reduce the efficacy of methotrexate in the treatment of acute lymphoblastic leukemia, which means that folic acid supplements could also reduce the efficacy of treatment of other cancers. Folic acid can have direct convulsant activity in some people, reversing the effects of the prescription drugs phenobarbital and primidone, and worsening seizure control.

Folic acid, in doses of 1 milligram per day or more, can reduce serum levels of phenytoin in some patients—as a result, increases in seizure frequency have been reported. Folic acid can antagonize the antiparasitic effects of pyrimethamine against Toxoplasmosis and Pneumocystis carinii pneumonia.

DOSAGE

The daily dosage for vitamin B_{12} should be about 500 micrograms. Folic acid should be taken in daily doses of 400 to 500 micrograms.

COMPLEMENTARY TREATMENTS

There are two complementary treatments that, when researched, stand out as effective in the treatment of diabetic retinopathy. These two treatments are acupuncture and magnet therapy. Both will be discussed in this section.

Acupuncture

Studies have shown that acupuncture, an ancient Chinese therapy involving inserting thin needles into various locations on the body, can be beneficial in the treatment of diabetic retinopathy.

In one study, one hundred and twenty individuals with diabetic retinopathy were randomly divided into an acupuncture group and a control group (sixty people per group). The acupuncture group was treated with the acupoints used for regulating the spleen and stomach, and the control group was treated with the acupoints around the eyes. In order to determine clinical therapeutic effect, researchers evaluated the acupuncture's effect on eye condition, blood glucose, blood lipids, nitric oxide (NO; a chemical messenger that helps dilate the blood vessels), and endothelin (ET; proteins that constrict blood vessels) levels. The needling method for regulating the spleen and stomach not only improved the retinopathy, but also helped regulate blood glucose, blood lipids, and NO and ET levels, with significant differences as compared with those in the control group.[19]

In another study, six hundred Chinese patients with clinically diagnosed retinopathy were treated by consecutive courses of acupuncture. After three months, 86 percent of the patients experienced normalization of their retinal fluid levels, a result similar to the natural history of the disease as reported by others in non-Chinese patients.[20]

In other research, thirty-two cases of retinal vein obstruction were treated by acupuncture and oral administration of

Chinese herbs.[21] The total effective rate was 90 percent, demonstrating significant effectiveness of the treatment.

Magnet Therapy

Magnet therapy is a complementary and alternative medicine practice involving the use of magnetic fields or electromagnetic radiation. In one study, magnets were attached on acupuncture points of diabetic retinopathy patients' outer ears.[22] This treatment not only lowered blood glucose levels, but improved eye conditions as well. Similarly, in a review of fifteen years of experimental and clinical research in magnetic therapy, the pain-relieving and regenerative effects of variable magnets were observed.[23] The influence of these fields on enzymatic and hormonal activity, free oxygen radicals, carbohydrates, protein, and lipid metabolism—as well as behavioral reactions and activity of dopamine receptors— was demonstrated.

Finally, clinical studies proved that magnet therapy and magnetostimulation (a noninvasive method to excite neurons in the brain through weak electric currents induced by rapidly changing magnetic fields) had high therapeutic efficacy in the treatment of several disorders, among them diabetic retinopathy.

CONCLUSION

Ignoring the signs of diabetic retinopathy can only lead to dire consequences. Additionally, failing to have your eyes checked simply because you do not have symptoms of diabetic retinopathy can also be detrimental, since the disease often progresses without any signs. Despite the high prevalence of retinopathy among diabetics, there is much that you can do to prevent it. Additionally, if you already have it, there is much you can do to prevent its worsening—you can even improve your vision.

By taking an active role in monitoring your condition and considering the use of one or more of the suggestions discussed in this chapter, you can make an important difference.

The next chapter will depart from discussions about nerve, circulatory, and cardiovascular health in diabetes, and will instead focus upon an issue of significant proportions: weight gain and loss.

CHAPTER 9

WEIGHT GAIN AND DIABETES

Being overweight is a contributing risk factor for the development of type-2 diabetes. Being obese is a *major* risk factor, especially if the weight was gained during adulthood. Obesity is measured by a person's body mass index (BMI). Having a BMI of 25 or greater represents obesity. (To learn how to measure your BMI, see Appendix D on page 181.)

If you are already diabetic, this information may not seem particularly important at this point in time. However, researchers have established that the amount of time a person remains overweight or obese is directly related to insulin concentration—and healthy insulin concentration is certainly important for diabetics to try to achieve.[1] Consequently, weight loss should be a major goal in the treatment strategy of an overweight diabetic—just as diabetics of average or normal weight should strive to maintain.[2]

The problem is that for most people, losing weight is not a particularly easy task. If you are hoping that this chapter will reveal some miraculous dietary supplement that will cause you to magically melt away pounds without diet and exercise, let me be very clear: it doesn't. Without dietary modification and exercise, weight loss is virtually impossible. That being said, there are definitely dietary supplements and complementary treatments that, when used along with diet and exercise, can help you achieve your weight loss goals quickly and efficiently. This chapter will discuss those supplements and treatments.

117

While Chapter 2 examined different dietary programs, this chapter will focus more on different options to lose weight, along with supplements and therapies that have been deemed both safe for diabetics and effective for weight loss. The chapter will start by examining the bottom line in weight loss, along with detailing a few diet support options. Next, it will take a look at some specific dietary supplements that may help promote weight loss. Finally, other complementary treatments, including exercise, that have been shown to be beneficial for weight loss will be explored.

DIETARY MODIFICATION: THE BOTTOM LINE IN WEIGHT LOSS

It has often been said that weight loss is simply an issue of calories in versus calories out—in other words, a balance between how many calories you eat and how many you burn up, implying that as long as you burn more calories than you eat, you will lose weight. While there is truth in this statement, it is also a gross oversimplification. The truth is, there are many variables, including genetic predisposition and metabolic tendency to store and burn fat, that determine how easy or difficult a time a person will have losing weight. In fact, chances are almost all of us know at least one person who seems to be able to eat as much as he or she wants without any adverse weight gain ramifications. There are biochemical reasons why this happens, but the bottom line is that for most of us it does not matter, since we are stuck losing weight the old-fashioned way: by watching our diet and getting enough exercise.

Since this book has already addressed the issue of diet, there is no point in reviewing the different diet programs again here. The same diet plans discussed in Chapter 2 are also beneficial for weight loss. If you have not already done so, take time now to read Chapter 2 (page 13). Additionally, Appendix A (see page 157) provides more detailed information about following a low-glycemic index diet plan.

DIET SUPPORT OPTIONS

Many people have difficulty following a diet plan on their own. When this occurs, there are options that can help you stick with the program. A few of those options are detailed in this section.

Computer Support

The internet is an extremely useful tool for research, information, and communication. Therefore, why not use it to your benefit when attempting to lose weight? There are quite a few computer-based, personal weight loss websites that offer dietary support and guidance. According to one research story, successful online programs are defined by a structured approach to modifying caloric intake, the use of cognitive-behavioral strategies such as self-monitoring, and individualized feedback and support.[3] Another review of studies on internet programs for weight loss found that most of the programs that were examined resulted in some degree of success in promoting weight loss.[4]

Of course, many people would agree that the less money these programs cost, the better. Luckily, when it comes to the internet, there are many free options available. One free internet support program can be found at the www.mypyramid.gov website under the "Interactive Tools" section. There, you can enter some data and the site will provide you with a general food group plan, a specific menu plan, and an online dietary and physical activity assessment tool that includes information on your diet quality, physical activity status, related nutrition messages, and links to information about nutrients and physical activity.

Consult with a Nutrition Professional

Nutritionists, dieticians, and weight loss doctors (bariatric physicians) can provide you with a personalized diet and weight loss program. Furthermore, regular visits to these nutritional professionals can help you to stay on track with your program. In one study, results showed that weekly consultations with a nutritionist for one year helped overweight subjects successfully lose weight and body fat. Moreover, the metabolic and cardiovascular risk markers—such as waist circumference, blood pressure, serum triglycerides, and blood glucose—declined significantly for these patients.[5]

Other research has shown similar results.[6] In a one-year, physician-directed program with dietician support, overweight subjects met with their physician initially, and then returned for follow-up visits at weeks four, twelve, twenty-four, thirty-six, and fifty-two. These patients had also consulted with a registered dietitian at weekly intervals for the first twelve weeks of the study, and then monthly for the remaining nine months. The results showed that the subjects successfully lost a significant amount of weight.[7]

To find a nutrition professional see Appendix B on page 169.

Join a Weight Loss Group

There are many weight loss group programs that offer support. Two such programs are Overeaters Anonymous (OA) and Weight Watchers International (WW). OA emphasizes the psychological and spiritual components of weight loss, with its main focus on commitment to the group. WW is also rooted in the fellowship of community, but adopts a model that is more focused on personal behavior. Although WW supplies more practical strategies for managing overeating, both groups provide a framework for developing positive, adaptive, and self-nurturing modalities.[8] Additionally, WW (along with some other popular programs) offers prepackaged meals that can be purchased either directly from the organization or in the frozen food section of your local supermarket.

Research has shown that individuals with eating disorders were able to successfully utilize OA skills and strategies.[9] Other research revealed that individuals with eating disorders found OA to be helpful in achieving their goals.[10]

In a study conducted on subjects participating in the WW program, the subjects experienced positive psychological changes and improved quality of life.[11] Furthermore, long-term assessment of individuals who lost weight following the WW plan showed that a large percentage were able to success-fully maintain their weight for a number of years.[12]

While OA and WW are not the only examples of weight loss group programs that offer support, they are certainly two that you may want to consider for yourself.

Personal Chef Services

For many people, finding the time to prepare and cook nutri-tious meals is a major roadblock when trying to follow an appropriate diet plan. Today, however, there are cooking serv-ices that will prepare meals and deliver them fresh to your home. Fortunately, these personal chef services are not always as expensive as one may think. In many cases, they prepare several complete meals in advance to your specifications, and put them in containers before delivering so that they are ready to eat when it is mealtime. Generally, the only time you need to factor in is heating up what these services have already made for you.

To find a personal chef near you, see Appendix B, begin-ning on page 169.

DIETARY SUPPLEMENTS

When it comes to possible dietary supplements that assist with weight loss, the sky is the limit. However, when it comes to well-researched dietary supplements that actually have some value, the playing field is remarkably smaller. The supplements that are discussed in this section are some of those with real value—that is, those with scientific studies to support their use. Please note that if you do not see a certain type of supplement listed here, it is not necessarily because it does not work (although that is a possibility). The reason a supplement may go unmentioned could be that it works but has health risks that I deem inappropriate for diabetics, or it may be that I just have not yet seen any good research on the supplement to warrant its inclusion in this chapter. In any case, the supplements I have chosen for this chapter include Caralluma fimbriata, Cissus quadrangularis, Coleus forskohlii, fish oil, and green tea.

Caralluma Fimbriata

Caralluma fimbriata is a plant used by tribal people in India to suppress hunger and enhance endurance.[13] As a standardized extract, Caralluma has been tested in human clinical studies and has been shown to have benefit for weight loss, reduced waist circumference, reduced appetite, or a combination of these. In a double-blind trial, Caralluma extract was assessed in fifty overweight men and women (twenty-five to sixty years old) for sixty days. All subjects were given standard advice regarding a weight-reducing diet and physical activity. Upon completion of the study, waist circumference and hunger levels showed a significant decline in the Caralluma group, compared to the placebo group.[14]

In another double-blind study of twenty-four overweight subjects (using the same dose of Caralluma as the previous study), 83 percent of the subjects lost weight, with 61 percent losing about six pounds. The highest recorded loss was nine pounds. Likewise, 72 percent of subjects reduced their waist by .5 to 3 inches, and 27 percent felt an increase in energy while taking standardized Caralluma extract.[15] In addition, the safety of Caralluma extract has been demonstrated in clinical research.[16]

Caralluma appears to be well-tolerated and has no known drug interactions.

DOSAGE

The dose used for the studies was 1 gram Caralluma extract per day (500 milligrams before two major meals).

Cissus Quadrangularis

Cissus quadrangularis (CQ) is an herb used in India to promote the fracture-healing process, as well as for other purposes in Ayurvedic medicine. It can also be helpful for diabetics who are looking to reduce their weight. In a double-blind, ten week study, seventy-two obese or overweight subjects received either two daily 150 milligram doses of CQ extract (standardized to 2.5 percent ketosteroids and 15 percent soluble plant fiber), two daily doses of a combination of CQ (150 milligrams) and the herb Irvingia gabonensis (250 milligrams) (together known as CQ/IG), or a placebo. All supplements were administered before meals.[17] Neither major dietary changes nor exercises were suggested during the study. Compared to the placebo group, the two active groups showed a statistically significant decrease in body weight, body fat, waist size, total plasma cholesterol, LDL cholesterol, and fasting blood glucose—all by week ten. For example, the CQ group reduced their percentage of body weight by almost 9 percent, compared to about a 2 percent reduction in the placebo group.

In a similar double-blind, six to eight week study, 150 overweight and obese persons received either two daily 150 milligram doses of CQ extract, two daily doses of a combination of CQ with other natural substances (CQ+), or a placebo.[18] Subjects were encouraged to maintain their normal levels of physical activity, and were also put on a calorie-restricted diet (2,100 calories a day). The results were that the CQ and CQ+ subjects experienced statistically significant reductions in weight, blood glucose levels, and serum lipids when compared to placebo group. For example, the CQ group lost almost nine pounds, while the placebo group lost only two and a half.

In a third double-blind study with 123 overweight and obese subjects using the same CQ+ combination, there were statistically significant net reductions in weight and central obesity, as well as in fasting blood glucose and serum lipids.[19]

Cissus quadrangularis appears to be well-tolerated, and has no known drug interactions.

DOSAGE

Two daily 150 milligram doses of CQ extract (standardized to 2.5 percent ketosteroids and 15 percent soluble plant fiber) is an appropriate amount for diabetics to use.

Coleus Forskohlii

Coleus (Coleus forskohlii) is an herb used in Ayurvedic medicine. Its active principle is known as forskolin. With regard to weight loss, Coleus has been shown to promote lipolysis (the breakdown of fat in the fat cells). In one open-label trial, six obese women were given 250 milligrams of Coleus (standardized for 10 percent forskolin) twice daily for eight weeks.[20] The women were asked to maintain previous daily physical exercise and eating habits. The results showed an average weight loss of 9.2 pounds, almost an 8 percent reduction in percentage of body fat, and a 4.2 percent increase in percentage of lean mass.

In an double-blind study, sixty obese volunteers who were given the same dose of Coleus as in the previous study experienced a significant decrease in average body weight compared to placebo (-3.8 pounds versus + .5 pounds), an average decrease in percent body fat compared to control (–.5 percent versus +.7 percent), and significant increases in lean body mass compared to the control.[21]

In another double-blind study, thirty overweight and obese men were given either the same dose of Coleus as in the previous studies or a placebo for twelve weeks.[22] The results were a significant decrease in body fat percentage (11.2 percent in the Coleus group compared to 1.7 percent in the placebo group) and almost a 6 percent increase in lean mass in Coleus group, while the placebo group had less than half the increase.

A twelve-week, open field trial on fourteen overweight and obese volunteers (thirteen women and one man), used a lower dose of 125 milligrams of Coleus (standardized for 10 percent forskolin) two times daily.[23] The results showed a statistically significant decrease in body weight and body fat.

In another twelve-week study (this one double-blind), nineteen mildly overweight women were given 250 milligrams of Coleus per day.[24] However, this study yielded different results. Neither the Coleus group nor the placebo group lost weight, although the Coleus group did experience less hunger and less fatigue. In addition, subjects taking the Coleus were successful at preventing weight gain.

In considering the studies, it appears that 250 milligrams of Coleus (standardized for 10 percent forskolin) given twice daily may be effective in the treatment of overweight and obese individuals, but not for mildly overweight individuals.

There have been no reports of adverse effects in oral administration of Coleus. Theoretically, concomitant use of Coleus and anticoagulant or antiplatelet agents might increase the risk of bruising and bleeding. Additionally, using Coleus with calcium channel blockers might cause additive coronary vasodilatory effects. Using Coleus with nitrates such as nitroglycerin and isosorbide might cause additive coronary vasodilatory effects.

DOSAGE

A good daily dose of Coleus (standardized for 10 percent forskolin) is 500 milligrams (250 milligrams twice a day).

Fish Oil

Research indicates fish oil intake from dietary fish sources improves weight loss and decreases blood glucose and insulin concentrations in overweight and hypertensive patients.[25] Double-blind, clinical research also shows that taking 6 grams a day of a fish oil supplement that provides the omega-3 fatty acids DHA (260 milligrams per gram) and EPA (60 milligrams per gram) significantly decreases body fat when combined with exercise.[26] In a randomized study, young, overweight men who included either lean fish, fatty fish, or fish oil (DHA/EPA capsules) as part of an energy-restricted diet lost approximately 2.2 pounds more after four weeks than those without including seafood or supplement of marine origin did.[27]

Additionally, in an open-label trial, six volunteers were fed a control diet (eating whatever they wanted) during a period of three weeks. Ten to twelve weeks later, the same volunteers were told to follow the same diet, but this time 6 grams daily of visible fat were replaced by 6 grams of fish oil. Again, the diet lasted three weeks. The results showed a statistically significant decrease in body fat mass with fish oils (almost 2 pounds) compared to no fish oils (less than 1 pound). The authors of the study concluded that fish oils reduce body fat mass and stimulate lipid oxidation in healthy adults.[28]

Furthermore, in a study published in the journal *Appetite*, researchers examined the effect of low dose (260 milligrams) and high dose (1,300 milligrams) omega-3 fatty acid supplements from fish oil and a low-calorie diet on appetite. The research focused on 232 overweight and obese volunteers.[29] The results were that subjects taking the high dose of omega-3 fatty acids had a reduction in hunger both directly after meals and two hours later. Blood analysis indicated that higher omega-3 fatty acids were associated with a reduction in appetite.

Orally, fish oils are generally well-tolerated at doses of 3 to 4 grams a day or less. Fish oil supplements can cause a fishy aftertaste or "fishy burp." Additionally, fish oils can lower blood pressure and might have additive effects in those treated with antihypertensives.

DOSAGE

For weight loss, a daily dose of fish oils should provide 1,560 milligrams DHA and 360 milligrams of EPA. For appetite control, 1,300 milligrams of omega-3 fatty acids (DHA and EPA combined) taken after meals should yield results.

Green Tea

Research has demonstrated that green tea is capable of stimulating thermogenesis and promoting fat oxidation (burning body fat). In a double-blind, three-day study, subjects who were given green tea providing 270 milligrams of catechins and 150 milligrams of caffeine daily experienced a significant increase in energy expenditure (calories burned).[30]

In an uncontrolled, open label, multicenter, three-month study, subjects given the same dose of green tea as the previous study decreased their body weight by 4.6 percent and their waist circumference by 4.5 percent.[31] In another double-blind, three-month study, subjects given the same dose of green tea found that after their initial weight loss, they were able to maintain their weight loss throughout the study.[32] This was only true, however, of habitual low caffeine consumers. Habitual high caffeine consumers receiving the green tea/caffeine mixture had no greater body weight maintenance than the high-caffeine group that received placebo. This is consistent with the results of another study in which green tea consumption after weight loss did not improve weight loss maintenance relative to the placebo group.[33] Thus, it can be assumed that a person's habitual caffeine intake plays a role in how effective supplementation with green tea will be for weight loss and weight maintenance.

High doses of green tea extract may cause gastrointestinal upset and/or central nervous system stimulation in some people. Additionally, the caffeine in green tea might increase the risk of additive central nervous system effects with amphetamines. The polyphenol catechins and caffeine in green tea are reported to have antiplatelet activity, so theoretically green tea might increase the risk of bleeding when used with antiplatelet or anticoagulant drugs (although this interaction has not been reported in humans).

DOSAGE

Green tea supplements are available in many potencies where the herbal extract is standardized for 20, 50, 60, or even 90 percent polyphenol catechins. So which potency should you get? The answer is that it doesn't matter, as long as you receive enough polyphenol catechins per dose. To ensure this, simply make sure the green tea product you choose provides you with a daily dose of 270 milligrams of polyphenol catechins. For example, if a green tea product were standardized for 60 percent polyphenol catechins, you would need 450 milligrams of catechins extract (270 divided by 0.60 = 450 milligrams). [To determine this, divide the required amount of catechins (270 milligrams) by the percentage of polyphenol catechins the product you are considering is standardized for (so 60 percent would equal .60). This will yield the dose of green tea you would need in order to get 270 milligrams of catechins. (In this case, 270 divided by .60 = 450.)

COMPLEMENTARY TREATMENTS

For weight loss, complementary treatments that have been shown to have good results include acupuncture, oxyhydro-massage, tai chi, and yoga. Of course, exercise is a mainstay of weight loss treatment.

The following section includes discussions of these complementary treatments and the role they play in weight loss.

Acupuncture

Acupuncture, which involves inserting thin needles into various points on the body, can help diabetics who need to lose weight. Research has demonstrated that acupuncture is effective in treating obesity with various methods, and without toxic side effects.[34] Studies have shown that acupuncture can affect appetite, intestinal motility, and metabolism, as well as emotional factors like stress.

Acupuncture increases neural activity in the hypothalamus (where appetite control hormones are made), in tone in the smooth muscle of the stomach. It has been observed that acupuncture application to obese people increases excitability of the satiety center in the hypothalamus, which helps people feel full and satisfied. Additionally, acupuncture stimulates the auricular branch of the vagal nerve and raises serotonin levels.

Both of these activities have been shown to increase tone in the smooth muscle of the stomach, thus suppressing appetite.

Among other things, serotonin enhances intestinal motility. It also controls stress and depression via endorphin and dopamine production. In addition to these effects, it is thought that the increase in plasma levels of beta endorphin after acupuncture application can contribute to weight loss in obese people by mobilizing stored body fat.[35,36]

Exercise

The importance of exercise in weight loss is universally understood and accepted, so there is no need to make the case for it here. However, not everyone is aware that exercising to lose weight does not have to consist of brutal sessions at the gym six times per week. Rather, something as simple as taking a brisk walk that lasts thirty to forty minutes, four or more times per week can help with weight loss.

In any case, to burn fat during exercise you must reach and sustain between 60 and 70 percent of your maximum target heart rate. This means that you must begin at a warm-up pace and move up to a faster pace, which will increase your heart rate. Be sure to spend the last three to five minutes of your workout at a slower pace for cool down. (To determine your target heart rate, see page 132.)

Oxyhydromassage

Both the consumption of oxygen-rich mineral water and hydromassage (applying massage techniques through the water) are methods used to increase oxygen levels in the human body without the benefit of the respiratory system (hyperoxygenisation). The combination of the two methods, called oxyhydromassage, was administered daily to fifty-seven overweight volunteers during a three-week treatment period. The results showed an average five pound loss of body weight and an average 3.2 percent decrease in body fat. Hyperoxygenisation occurred in 68 to 75 percent of the participants. The researchers presumed that the hyperoxygenisation effect accelerated the oxidative (aerobic) activity in mitochondria of the muscles, the site at which fat is burned as fuel.[37]

Tai Chi

Tai Chi is a graceful form of exercise that has existed for centuries. A blind, randomized experimental trial examined the therapeutic effect of a multidisciplinary weight management program by incorporating Tai Chi exercises among twenty-one sedentary obese women with medical providers. All subjects participated in a ten-week weight management program that included a low-calorie, balanced diet; a weekly physician/psychologist/dietician group session; and an exercise program. For the exercise component, subjects were randomized to either a two-hour weekly session of Tai Chi or a conventional structured exercise program. The results showed that the Tai Chi group improved in resting systolic blood pressure, chair-rise test (to measure leg strength), mood, and reduced percent of fat at week ten and at a six month follow-up. General self-efficacy was enhanced in both groups and was maintained at thirty weeks.[38]

Yoga

Yoga is a combination of breathing exercises, physical postures, and meditation aimed at training the consciousness to promote control of the body and mind. In an uncontrolled, open study, yoga's effect on the weight of children and adolescents at risk for developing type-2 diabetes was investigated. Secondarily, the impact of yoga on self-concept and psychiatric symptoms was measured. The results were that after twelve

Finding Your Maximum Target Heart Rate

To burn fat, you must reach and sustain between 60 and 70 percent of your maximum target heart rate during exercise.

One method used to find what 60 percent of your maximum target heart rate would be is based on the number of times the heart beats per minute during or immediately following exercise.

- To determine 60 percent of your maximum target heart rate, follow these steps.

   1. Subtract your age from 220.

   2. Multiply that number by 60 percent to yield beats per minute.

   3. Divide the result by 6.

This will give you your 60 percent maximum target rate for a ten second period.

- To find what 70 percent of your maximum target rate, follow these steps.

   1. Subtract your age from 220.

   2. Multiply that number by 70 percent to yield beats per minute.

   3. Divide the result by 6.

This will give you your 70 percent maximum target rate for a ten second period.

For example, a thirty-six-year-old's equation for 60 percent maximum target heart rate would look like this:

$$220 - 36 = 184; 184 \times .6 = 110 \text{ beats per minute;}$$
$$110 \div 6 = 18.33 \text{ beats per ten seconds.}$$

This is the 60 percent maximum target heart rate.

The same person's 70 percent maximum target heart rate equation would look like this:

$$220 - 36 = 184; 184 \times .7 = 128.8 \text{ beats per minute};$$
$$128.8 \div 6 = 21.4 \text{ beats per ten seconds.}$$

Therefore, when calculating target heart rate to burn fat, this person's should fall between 18 and 21 (60 and 70 percent).

Once you know where your heart rate *should* fall, see where it does fall. Immediately following exercise, watch the second hand on a clock. Place your fingers on a pressure point on the neck or wrist, and count the number of times your heart beats within ten seconds. The number should fall between your high and low maximum target heart rate numbers. If it does, this will ensure your body is effectively burning fat. Preferably, you should be at the high end of these numbers, but anywhere in between is fine.

An easier way to calculate your target heart rate was proposed by exercise physiologist Covert Bailey, in his book, *The New Fit or Fat:*

". . . try singing 'God Bless America'. If you can't get beyond the first word without gasping for air, you're exercising too hard. On the other hand, if you get past 'land that I love', before you need your first breath, you should speed up."[39]

The best exercises that allow you to reach your target heart rate are aerobic exercises. Examples of aerobic exercises that are good for burning fat are:

- Aerobics class
- Bike riding
- Brisk walking
- Jogging
- Roller skating/blading
- Swimming

weeks, the average weight loss was 4.4 pounds. Furthermore, four out of five children with low self-esteem experienced improvement in the area, and overall anxiety symptoms improved as well.[40] Weight loss results with yoga therapy were seen in other research as well.[41]

CONCLUSION

My hope is that this chapter has provided you with useful strategies to help you in the battle of the bulge. Additionally, trying one of the diets discussed in Chapter 2 will also help, especially when paired with one of the techniques in this chapter. Utilize diet support options as needed. Incorporate some type of exercise program into your lifestyle. Take one or more of the dietary supplements discussed. Consider trying one of the complementary therapies.

You will discover that few changes in your life can have as dramatic an effect on so many areas of your health as weight loss can. For diabetics, this is doubly true. Weight loss can improve insulin resistance, reduce the risk of cardiovascular disease, reduce the risk of some types of cancer, and finally, help you feel better about yourself. You *can* make a difference in your life, and I hope this chapter has shown you just how significant that difference can be.

CHAPTER 10

HOW TO CHOOSE AND USE DIETARY SUPPLEMENTS

The hunt for the right supplement can be a confusing and intimidating process for anyone—especially for people who have not purchased or used supplements on a regular basis. If you are considering taking any of the supplements in this book, you likely have a lot of questions. I hope that this chapter will answer some of the main ones, thus making your transition into the world of supplements a bit easier.

The easiest way to find what you are looking for is to first understand what to look for, and to then ask the right questions if you can't find what you need. After all, there are a myriad of brands and products to search through. But what should you be looking for? What questions should you ask? Read on and find out.

In this chapter, you will find the common questions people have about dietary supplements. The information after each question is designed to provide you with some guidelines for wading through the confusing mass of dietary supplement labels. Additionally, you will gain knowledge about choosing and using the products that are most likely to meet your needs.

The format of this chapter is a bit different from the other chapters in the book. It has been organized into a simple question-and-answer format, with a few charts and insets added where appropriate. I hope this makes it easy for you to locate answers to any questions you may have.

135

Why should I take more nutrients than suggested by the government?

Over the years, governmental dietary allowances and standards have been frequently revised and renamed. For the purposes of labeling, it began with the Minimum Daily Requirements (MDR) in 1941. The primary goal of the MDR was to prevent diseases caused by nutrient deficiencies. It was originally intended to evaluate and plan for the nutritional adequacy of groups—for example, the armed forces and children in school lunch programs—rather than to determine the nutrient needs of individuals.

In 1973, the FDA established a new standard called the United States Recommended Daily Allowances (U.S. RDA) for use in nutrition labeling. The U.S. RDA replaced the MDR, which had been used since 1941, in the labeling of food and dietary supplements. The U.S. RDA was deemed to be the amount of various nutrients needed by healthy people, plus an additional 30 to 50 percent to allow for individual variations. For example, if 1 milligram of vitamin B_1 was deemed to be adequate, then increasing it by 50 percent to 1.5 milligrams was considered optimal to allow for individual variations. Nevertheless, it can be argued that this "one-size-fits-all" nutrient standard is not really the best way to establish the nutrient needs for a diverse population.

Then, in 1994, the Daily Value (DV) was created. Essentially, the DV is exactly the same as the U.S. RDA, with a couple of new minerals. The DV is the current governmental standard.

What each of these standards has in common is they represent the amount of a vitamin or mineral a person should consume daily to prevent a deficiency disease. However, many nutrition experts argue that while taking in the DV of a vitamin or mineral is enough to prevent a deficiency disease, the same amount is totally inadequate for modern lifestyle needs and disease prevention. For example, the DV for vitamin C is 60 milligrams, which would help prevent the classic vitamin C deficiency disease known as "scurvy." However, research has shown that taking 300 milligrams of vitamin C a day (5 times the DV) can decrease the risk of death from cardiovascular diseases by 42 percent in men and 25 percent in women.[1] Consequently, it often makes sense to consume vitamins in levels that exceed the DV. When it comes to minerals, however, the DV amounts are generally right on track for general health needs and disease prevention.

An alternative recommendation for vitamins is the optimal daily intake (ODI), a term coined by nutritionist Shari Lieberman, PhD.[2] The ODI is based upon the results of published research, which demonstrate a clear benefit for most people in regard to consuming higher levels of vitamins and minerals than indicated in the DV. See Tables 10.1 and 10.2 on pages 138 and 139 for my ODI recommendations, as compared to DV.

Additionally, sometimes exceeding the ODI levels can be beneficial. Instances when this is the case are discussed throughout this book in the supplement recommendations. For example, taking up to 1,000 micrograms of chromium daily has been shown to be beneficial for diabetics, even though the DV and ODI are 120 micrograms.[3]

What is the difference between natural and synthetic ingredients?

To understand the difference between natural and synthetic ingredients, we should first define the terms "natural" and "synthetic." Unfortunately, there is not one definitive way to do this. Some people say that whether a vitamin is natural or synthetic depends on its source. Based on this fundamentalist position, vitamins that originate from food or plant sources are

Table 10.1	Recommended ODI for Vitamins	
Vitamin	**DV**	**OTI**
Biotin	300 micrograms	300 micrograms
Choline	Not established	40 to 100 milligrams
Folate	400 micrograms	400 to 800 micrograms
Niacin (Vitamin B_3)	20 milligrams	40 to 100 milligrams (as niacinamide)
Pantothenic Acid	10 milligrams	40 to 100 milligrams
Riboflavin (Vitamin B_2)	1.7 milligrams	40 to 100 milligrams
Thiamin (Vitamin B_1)	1.5 milligrams	40 to 100 milligrams
Vitamin A	5,000 international units	10,000 international units (as beta-carotene)
Vitamin B_6	2 milligrams	40 to 100 milligrams
Vitamin B_{12}	6 micrograms	40 to 100 micrograms
Vitamin C	60 milligrams	1,000 to 3,000 milligrams
Vitamin D	400 international units	1,000 to 2,000 international units
Vitamin E	30 international units	400 to 800 international units
Vitamin K	80 micrograms	80 micrograms

natural, while vitamins created in a laboratory are synthetic. In other words, the vitamin C found in a fresh glass of orange juice would be considered to be natural vitamin C.

Others believe that the chemical form of a vitamin (whether the molecule has a left rotation, designated as "L", or a right rotation, designated as "D") is the factor that dictates whether it is natural or synthetic. For example, since the chemical form of vitamin C found in orange juice is L-ascorbic acid (the sci-

Table 10.2	Recommended ODI for Minerals	
Mineral	**DV**	**OTI**
Calcium	1,000 milligrams	1,000 to 1,500 milligrams
Chromium	120 micrograms	120 micrograms
Copper	2 milligrams	2 milligrams
Iodine	150 micrograms	150 micrograms
Iron	18 milligrams	18 milligrams
Magnesium	400 milligrams	400 to 750 milligrams
Manganese	2 milligrams	2 milligrams
Molybdenum	75 micrograms	75 micrograms
Phosphorus	1,000 milligrams	1,000 milligrams
Selenium	70 micrograms	70 micrograms
Zinc	15 milligrams	15 to 30 milligrams

entific name for vitamin C), then L-ascorbic acid would be considered natural even though it was created in a laboratory using corn syrup as the starting point. In my opinion, this second definition is more meaningful, and therefore, this is the definition that will be used for the purpose of this text.

To illustrate this point further, consider the following. A cup of freshly-squeezed orange juice will provide you with about 124 milligrams of vitamin C.[4] If you were able to cause all the liquid in the orange juice to evaporate—without destroying the heat and light-sensitive vitamin C—and then put the remaining powder into a capsule, you would still only get a little over 100 milligrams of "natural" (according to the first definition) vitamin C. If you wanted to take at least 1,000 milligrams a day, you would have to take about ten capsules, which is not practical. On the other hand, you could easily get

1,000 milligrams of vitamin C in a single tablet. However, to do that, the vitamin C would need to be derived from ascorbic acid that originated from the conversion of corn syrup to glucose. Additional enzymatic steps in the laboratory would need to be taken to ultimately yield purified, crystallized vitamin C. For those who believe in the second definition of natural, this form of vitamin C would still classify.

So, to answer the question, sometimes there is a significant difference between natural and synthetic. For example, natural vitamin E (d-alpha tocopherol/yl) is better utilized than synthetic vitamin E (dl-alpha tocopherol/yl). A 1981 study published in *The American Journal of Clinical Nutrition* demonstrated that natural vitamin E was 3.5 times more active in the human body than synthetic vitamin E, even though the same number of international units were used in the test subjects.[5] However, most times there is not a significant difference between natural and synthetic, at least when vitamins are concerned.

However, most B vitamins can only be made synthetically, with no natural alternative. Consequently, the argument is academic in the case of using synthetic B vitamins. If you decided that you wanted only natural vitamins, you would have to prepare yourself to accept the fact that there is almost no way you will be able to achieve high intakes of virtually any B vitamin in supplemental form.

Sticking with the second definition of natural, in the case of amino acids, you can tell whether or not they are natural by the "L" designation in found of the front of their name (such as L-carnitine). Most commercial amino acids are derived from the microbial fermentation of beet sugar. This "L" rule, however, does not hold true for all supplements. For example, in a previous paragraph about vitamin E, the D-form designates a natural produce.

Whole Food Vitamins

Are whole food vitamins all-natural? Not if you subscribe to the fundamentalist definition of natural. If you find this hard to believe, just go to the website of almost any company selling "whole food" vitamins and carefully read how these vitamins are created. Initially, the marketing copy on these websites generally present the vitamins as coming from a whole food, not chemical isolates. As a matter of fact, one website touts that their products do not contain "the synthetic vitamins, minerals and chemical herbal isolates you will find in most supplements."[6] However, when you further examine the process, you will learn that the distained, isolated, and synthetic vitamins are simply mixed together with whole foods in a type of broth, or more eloquently stated, "cultured in organic media."[7] The finished vitamins are then said to be delivered "in their safest and most active form within the infinite complexity of whole food."[8]

To sum up: Just because synthetic vitamins are mixed with whole foods, it does not make them a natural, whole food source.

Additionally, questions have been raised about whether whole food vitamins are all-natural. See the inset above for more information.

What is a standardized ingredient?

Standardized ingredients, particularly in the case of herbs, are an important part of the world of dietary supplements. You may have noticed that throughout this book when doses for certain supplements are given, the term "standardized" is used to designate a specific percentage of some component found in an herb or other ingredient. Naturally, this raises the question of what standardized means.

Well, all standardized really means is that the supplement, typically an herb, has been analyzed in a laboratory, and that it has been verified to contain a certain percentage of an active constituent or compound that is naturally found in that particular herb. For example, the active constituents in the herb milk thistle are collectively referred to as "silymarin." In the case of a good milk thistle extract, the herb will be standardized to provide 80 percent silymarin by weight. If, on the other hand, the herb was not standardized or was standardized for a lower percentage of silymarin, it can be assumed that the effectiveness of the herb will be significantly less.

The natural constituents and compounds that make up an herb can vary depending on how, where, and when the herb is grown. Having a standardized herb guarantees consumers that they are getting a consistent quality product, and can probably expect the same results from one batch to another.

In some cases, the compound being measured may be an active component in the herb, and in other cases it is just an easily identifiable marker used to determine quality. In either case, standardized herbs have the advantage of being natural medicines with reproducible effects every time they are consumed. Conversely, if an herb isn't standardized, you would not know if it provided a consistent amount of its active components from batch to batch, and you would not necessarily experience the same results every time you consumed it.

Whenever using herbs, I recommend standardized herbs for consistency and quality. However, there are two exceptions to the rule. One is if studies on an herb were conducted on a non-standardized herb. In that case, it would be acceptable to use the herb in its non-standardized form. The other exception is Chinese herbs used in traditional Chinese medicine. Chinese herbs have been used for thousands of years without any standardization.

How should supplements be stored?

Supplements should be stored in a cool, dry place—ideally, a cabinet in your kitchen—but not one to close to the stove or oven, which could result in heat exposure. Do not store them in your bathroom medicine cabinet, because the humidity from taking a bath or shower will work its way into the bottle, potentially ruining the tablets or capsules.

If you have probiotic products (such as Lactobacillus acidophilus), you should store them in your refrigerator to help extend their shelf life. This is because probiotics are live, viable microorganisms. Since vitamins and minerals are not alive, they do not need to be refrigerated.

How long will a dietary supplement last on the shelf?

If you have purchased your supplements from a good company, the product labels should provide an expiration date. The date will let you know how long the active ingredients—vitamins, minerals, herbs, etc.—in the product will be good for. You should always stick to this date—and if you still have some of the supplement left after its expiration, throw it out. If there is no expiration date, then switch to another brand.

If switching brands seems like an extreme recommendation, consider the fact that some supplements are manufactured and stored at the manufacturing facility for months—sometimes for over a year. Then, these supplements are shipped to the vitamin companies for whom they were manufactured, only to sit on their shelves for months. By the time they are shipped to distributors and placed on shelves that consumers can purchase them from, they may be well into their second or third year. If there is no expiration date on the product label, you have no idea how old the product is. This is a real problem, since many vitamin formulas have a twenty-four month shelf life. Why take a chance? Only purchase dietary supplements that have expiration dates.

How and when should I take my supplements?

How to take a supplement depends upon what the supplement is. As a rule of thumb, most vitamin and mineral formulas are best taken with a meal. The reason for this is that the presence of food stimulates digestion, which allows many vitamins and minerals to break down efficiently for absorption. B vitamins in particular can be a little rough on your stomach without any food present to dilute them, and sometimes consuming them on an empty stomach results in mild nausea.

Herbal products, on the other hand, are generally best taken between meals or on an empty stomach. The reason for this is, unlike vitamins and minerals, you don't want food to dilute them. With herbs, you'd like them to reach the intestines as soon as possible so they can be absorbed. Likewise, isolated amino acid products are generally best taken on any empty stomach, for the same reason. Other types of nutraceuticals, such as fish oils, should be taken with meals, since they can cause an upset stomach when taken without food.

When you should take your supplement also depends on the type of supplement you are taking. In general, supplements containing B vitamins (such as multivitamins) can make you feel energetic. Consequently, you probably would want to take these with breakfast or lunch, rather than with dinner, which could potentially keep you awake when you want to go to bed. If you are taking a supplement for general health purposes, you may want to spread out your dosage. Taking it in the morning and the evening allows you to maintain more consistent blood levels of the nutraceutical. However, for some products, dosage times are more obvious. For example, you should take a product formulated to help induce sleep about one hour before bedtime, and digestive enzymes should be taken with meals.

Table 10.3 is a good rule of thumb to follow for how and when to take supplements.

Table 10.3 How and When to Take Supplements		
Supplement	**How to Take**	**When to Take**
Adaptogenic herbs (Ginseng, Rhodiola, Ashwagandha)	On an empty stomach	Upon arising in the morning
Amino acids	On an empty stomach	Anytime
B Vitamins	With a meal	Breakfast or lunch
Herbs	On an empty stomach	Ideally, twice daily
Multivitamin	With a meal	Breakfast or lunch
Other nutraceuticals	With a meal	Ideally, breakfast and dinner
Probiotics	On an empty stomach	Once daily
Vitamins or minerals	With a meal	Ideally, breakfast and dinner

Keep in mind these guidelines are not carved in stone. You may very well find that a variation to this schedule works best for you.

Are some forms of supplements better absorbed than others?

The short answer to this question is yes, some forms of supplements are absorbed better than others. Sometimes this matters and sometimes it does not. In some cases, better absorption means you will receive more of the supplement's active ingredient—if you don't receive more, then greater absorption has limited appeal. Coenzyme Q-10 is a good example of when absorption rate matters. Research has shown that coenzyme Q-10 is better absorbed as an oil base in a softgel capsule than as a tablet or two-piece hardshell capsule. When taken as an oil base, the body received more coenzyme Q-10.[9]

On the contrary, an example of when absorption rate may not matter is calcium. Consider that calcium carbonate (the most common form of calcium used in supplements) has gotten a bad rap. Some have accused it of not being absorbed well, while others have indicated that alternative forms of calcium are actually better absorbed. In any case, calcium does not naturally exist by itself. Rather, it is attached to some type of organic or inorganic acid. Minerals attached to acids are called "mineral salts." All forms of calcium used in dietary supplements provide one or more calcium salts. For example, if you attached citric acid to calcium, you would have a calcium salt called calcium citrate (which is frequently touted as being a well absorbed form of calcium). The issue with different calcium salts is that they all provide different percentages of actual, or elemental, calcium by weight. Sticking with the example of calcium citrate, it provides about 22 percent elemental calcium.

By comparison, calcium carbonate is about 38 to 40 percent elemental calcium—a much higher elemental potency, and clearly a good source of calcium. What this means is that in order to obtain 500 milligrams of elemental calcium, you would have to consume either 2,273 milligrams of calcium citrate or 1,282 milligrams of calcium carbonate. If you used the same amount of calcium citrate and calcium carbonate, say 1,282 milligrams of each, you would receive more calcium from the carbonate. Even though citrate has a 13 percent greater absorption rate, you would still end up with far more calcium from the carbonate source.

The bottom line is that while some calcium salts are better absorbed than others, what is most important is to get the correct elemental amount of the mineral and to make sure to take the mineral supplement with a meal so that the hydrochloric acid in your stomach will break it down efficiently for absorption.

If you ever hear or read that a certain form of a nutrient is better absorbed, always ask your self the questions, "Is there proof?" and "Does the better absorbed form provide enough of the nutrient to do *me* any good?" Answering these will help you decide for your particular case how much the form the supplement is taken in matters.

Why does a dietary supplement need other ingredients?

The manufacturing of dietary supplements is a complex process. For example, in order to form the active ingredients in a multivitamin (vitamins, minerals, etc.) into a tablet and remain that way, it is necessary to add ingredients to the product that will bind the active ingredients together, and yet at the same time, release them during digestion. The tablet must be firm enough to withstand the rigors of handling during the processes of coating, packaging, and shipping, but it cannot be too firm or it will not break down completely in the digestive tract.

In addition, tablets have a tendency to become affected by mechanical problems during manufacturing, which can cause pieces of the tablet to fall off or get stuck in the tablet-punch machinery. All of this requires additives to be incorporated into the mix in order to prevent manufacturing problems, while still making the tablet an effective product for the customers' needs. Additionally, capsules have unique challenges that require specific additives to facilitate the manufacturing process.

Just below the "Supplement Facts" box on the label of a dietary supplement is a listing of "other ingredients." These other ingredients are the additives that help keep the tablet or capsule together, or in some way facilitate the manufacturing process. Without these other ingredients, there would be no tablet or capsule.

Is it better to use one ingredient or a combination of ingredients to address a health issue?

In most cases, a combination of ingredients is always the better option to treat a health issue. The reason for this is that sometimes ingredients work better when paired with other ingredients than they do on their own. For example, it doesn't matter how much calcium you take—it will not be absorbed unless you have a sufficient amount of vitamin D present. This type of synergistic relationship is especially common with vitamins and minerals, and illustrates the importance of using combinations of ingredients.

Complementary relationships between ingredients are another reason to utilize combinations. For example, a dietary supplement formulated to help lower cholesterol levels might include one ingredient that reduces the amount of cholesterol produced by the liver. It might also include another ingredient that interferes with the absorption of dietary fat or cholesterol in the intestines. A third ingredient may not lower cholesterol levels, but may increase HDL ("good" cholesterol) levels, which in turn may improve the balance of blood lipids.

By using a combination of different ingredients, it is often possible to achieve better results. In addition, combination formulas are generally more cost effective than purchasing ingredients individually.

Does a product that costs more have greater quality?

Sometimes cost is indicative of quality—but it is up to you to know what you are looking for and be a smart shopper. Buying the cheapest product may be a bad idea since it could reflect inferior ingredients and substandard manufacturing practices. Buying the most expensive product, however, does not necessarily mean that you are getting the highest-quality product. For example, if you purchase a product from a multi-level marketing company, the product is almost always overpriced since the distributor, supervising distributor, regional distributor, and so on all have to get a share of the profit. This does not mean that the multi-level marketing product is not good, it just means that you are likely going to pay a lot more for it than you would for its counterpart at a retail store.

In other cases, price can indeed be an indicator of quality. For example, if you are paying a higher price for a probiotic product, it may be because it cost more to manufacture and store the product under refrigerated conditions to maintain the viability of its microorganisms. A very cheap probiotic product, on the other hand, may not contain any live microorganisms.

What it often comes down to is how comfortable you are with the brand you have purchased. If the product is from a trustworthy brand, the chances are very good that you are getting a quality product.

How are the nutrients in supplements measured?

The way a nutrient is measured depends on what the nutrient is. Most water soluble vitamins (B and C vitamins), minerals, and amino acids are typically measured in milligrams. There are 1,000 milligrams in 1 gram. However, some vitamins and minerals, such as biotin, folic acid, vitamin B_{12}, chromium, and selenium are required in such small amounts that they must be measured in micrograms. There are 1,000 micrograms in 1 milligram, and 1,000,000 micrograms in 1 gram. Milligrams and micrograms are both measures of weight.

Conversely, the biological activity (the level of effectiveness in the body) of a fat soluble vitamin (A, D, and E vitamins) is expressed in terms of International Units (IU). It is not expressed in milligrams, because the IU can change based on the source of the vitamin. For example, 1 milligram of natural vitamin E has more IU of biological activity than 1 milligram of synthetic vitamin E. Therefore, the amount of a synthetic vitamin E product must be increased to reach the equivalent number of IU found in a natural vitamin E product. For this reason, fat soluble vitamins must be expressed in terms of IU.

How much you take of any supplement is important. Understanding the amount of what you are taking can be crucial in helping you reach your goal. When you read any label, you will see the amount of ingredients contained in each capsule or table. By understanding these measurements, you will be able to make better decisions about what to take.

Which is best, capsules, tablets, or liquids?

Whether you take your supplement in capsule, tablet, or liquid form depends upon what type of supplement you are buying, as well as your personal preferences. If you want high doses of a nutrient and do not want to take a lot of capsules, tablets are a good choice because you can fit more of a specific nutrient in a tablet than you can in a capsule. If you want a supplement to digest very quickly, a capsule is a good choice. Many herbal products are put in capsule form, since a rapid breakdown and exposure to stomach acid may be necessary to obtain certain active components from the herb.

Often, liquid supplements are touted as being superior because they are available for immediate absorption. While this may be true, it is not always an advantage. For example, if you take a liquid multivitamin with a meal, none of the nutrients it contains will be absorbed until the food passes through the stomach and reaches the intestines—so there is no real advantage in this case. Furthermore, it is hard to maintain nutrient stability in liquid supplements. A good example of this is liquid creatine (a muscle enhancing supplement). In a liquid form, the creatine is rapidly converted into creatinine, which has no muscle-enhancing value. That means you are better off taking creatine as a powder or tablet.

However, many people have trouble swallowing pills. If you fall into this category, a liquid supplement may be your best (and only) choice. Also, liquid extracts can be effective dosage forms for medicinal herbs—of course, the solid herbal extracts in capsule form are also effective.

How do I know what I'm getting?

Caveat emptor is Latin for "let the buyer beware," a policy that is always beneficial to follow. Being an aware buyer, how do you know that what is listed on the label is actually what is in the bottle? The unfortunate answer is you cannot know for sure. You can, however, increase your chances of buying a reputable product by making sure to limit your purchases to brands that you trust.

Naturally, the next question is how do you know what brands to trust? There are a few ways you can ascertain trustworthy brands. One is to check Appendix B of this book (page 169), in which I have listed a number of dietary supplement brands which, in my three decades of experience in the dietary supplement industry, I have found to be reputable. Another way is to talk to people who know the brands—specifically, talk to people who are in the business of selling supplements, such as those who work in vitamin stores or offices that sell supplements. Finally, when deciding what brands you can trust, you can find out if the manufacturer who makes the brand in question is GMP certified.

What does "GMP certified" mean?

The current Good Manufacturing Practice (cGMP) regulations enforced by the FDA provide for systems that assure proper design, monitoring, and control of manufacturing processes and facilities. Adherence to cGMP regulations assures the identity, strength, quality, and purity of dietary supplement products by requiring that manufacturers adequately control manufacturing operations.[10,11]

There are two recognized agencies that offer GMP certification. These include the Natural Products Association (NPA) and NSF International (NSF). Dietary supplement manufacturers who pass an extensive auditing process are awarded GMP certification from either NPA or NSF. Possession of GMP certification is verification that the manufacturer is generally in compliance with the FDA's cGMP. However, if a manufacturer does not have GMP certification it does not necessarily mean that it is not in compliance with cGMP—it is just more difficult to verify compliance. If this is the case, you may have to use one of the other methods discussed to ensure you are using a brand you can trust.

What all this means is that when you are looking for a brand of dietary supplements to purchase, try to look for one that has been manufactured in a GMP-certified manufacturing facility. In some cases, the label of the product will have a logo or statement indicating the GMP certification status. Unfortunately, this is not always the case. If GMP certification is not indicated on the bottle, you can contact the dietary supplement company and ask them if their products have been manufactured in a GMP-certified facility, and if so, by whom were they certified. You can also visit the websites for NPA and NSF (see the Resources section beginning on page 169) and see if the manufacturer or brand is listed.

From whom can I get reliable advice about dietary supplements?

Unfortunately, there is no consistent across-the-board answer for whom you can trust for dietary advice. In some cases, people who own vitamin stores are very knowledgeable and can offer reliable and trustworthy advice. But, there are many other cases in which retail salespeople give out bad or incorrect information. Some independent store owners and small retail vitamin chains provide their employees some training and/or education to help assure that they will make good recommendations to the retail customers (see Appendix B, page 169), but depending on circumstances you cannot always count on this.

In some cases, you will come across healthcare professionals who sell and/or recommend dietary supplements as part of their practice. Such individuals tend to make it their business to learn a great deal about dietary supplements. Licensed, naturopathic physicians in particular tend to have a significant knowledge of dietary supplements. Likewise, quite a few chiropractors have had coursework in the use of supplements. In addition, some nutritionists in private practices also have an expertise in the area. Appendix B will provide you with a listing of where you can find such healthcare professionals.

I encourage you to learn as much as you can about dietary supplements. Reading this book is a positive step in that direction, but there are other things you can do too. For a list of ways to become more familiar with supplements, see the Resources section (page 169).

Your aunt, co-worker, friend, or a random stranger are not the people to rely on for dietary supplement advice. They may have told you about something they took that worked for them, but that does not mean it will work for you, nor is it likely that any of these people have any real knowledge about dietary supplements beyond what they may have read in a magazine article or experienced firsthand. Although it is perfectly reasonable to love and respect these people in your life (with the possible exception of the random stranger), it does not make any sense to rely on their dietary supplement recommendations, however well-intentioned they may be.

CONCLUSION

Between the information provided in this chapter and the resources offered in Appendix B, you should now know enough to make some informed choices about buying and using dietary supplements. Also, do not be afraid to ask questions of people who are knowledgeable about dietary supplements if you need some help.

I can promise you this: the more you go out there, look around, and purchase these products, the less intimidated you will be. And the more questions you ask, the more you will learn. Remember, unless you actually take dietary supplements, you will never have an opportunity to benefit from them.

CONCLUSION

Diabetes afflicts millions of people, and if statistics are correct, that number will keep on growing. I wrote this book because I wanted to offer something that would really be able to help people. My hope was that by explaining how to use the many supplements and complementary therapies found in this book to help treat diabetes and their most common complications, many diabetics would learn to help themselves.

Now that you have read this book, what are you going to do with your newfound knowledge? What you decide to do next can make all the difference in the world. Doing nothing will mean that reading this book was a waste of your time—but I'm sure you want to feel better, and I really want you to as well. Now, you absolutely have the power to make it happen. This book gives many examples of places to start. It is up to you to choose one and more forward from there.

As you work toward improving your condition, it is extremely important for you to remember that this book is meant to be an *adjunct* to a diabetic's existing diet and drug program, *not* a replacement for that program. To that end, it is vital that you work with a physician or healthcare professional when following any of the suggestions or recommendations in this book.

The reasons you should work with a physician vary, but they are nonetheless important. For one, you may become a victim of your own success. What I mean by this is your blood glucose levels may indeed drop. Additionally, if you are currently using insulin, the amount of insulin that your body requires may also drop. If this happens, your physician *must* be aware because the dosage of your medication may need to be adjusted. In most cases, this will not be too difficult since you will generally be testing your blood glucose before determining the appropriate insulin dose. However, for those who use an oral hypoglycemic medication (a pill), this becomes more problematic because you cannot adjust the dosage. In this instance, it is particularly important that you work closely with your physician so that adjustments can be made to your medication accordingly.

Additionally, your physician is most likely aware of all your health problems, current and former. It is possible that he or she may know of some legitimate reason that you should avoid a certain supplement or complementary therapy practice. Only by sharing your plans with your physician can he or she advise you accordingly.

It is time for you to take control of your diabetes and your health. It is time to prevent complications, or further complications, that arise as a result of your diabetes. It is time to do something. Take the next step by taking power over your diabetes. Choose a program, speak with your physician, and get started.

As you progress through your chosen program, I would love to hear your stories of success. Additionally, if you have any questions about the book—or about diabetes in general—I would love to hear those too. You can send me any questions, comments, or success stories in email form to gbruno@hchs.edu.

APPENDIX A

FOLLOWING A LOW GLYCEMIC INDEX DIET

In Chapter 2 (page 13), the concept of a low glycemic index (GI) diet was introduced. This appendix provides some additional information about the rationale for this diet, as well as some direction on how to personalize a low glycemic index diet for yourself—and how to follow it.

THE SLOW-CARB DIET

In a study from the *American Journal of Clinical Nutrition*, a slow carbohydrate or "slow-carb" diet focusing on low-glycemic index foods was found to be far more effective than traditional low-carb, low-fat, or low-calorie diets for losing weight and preventing heart disease (both of which can be complications associated with diabetes).[1-3] In the study, eleven obese young adults did not avoid carbs or fats, nor did they count calories or eat prepackaged foods. Despite this, these slow-carb dieters lost more weight than twelve of their peers on a conventional low-fat diet. In addition, the slow-carb dieters lowered their risk of heart disease. Furthermore, they achieved all of this while still eating plenty of satisfying foods.

The slow-carb diet focused on low GI foods, and appeared to be easier to follow than diets restricted in either fat or carbs. The base of the GI diet is to eat plenty of fruits and vegetables cooked or served with healthful oils. Next are reduced-fat dairy foods; lean meats and fish; nuts; and beans. Following, and meant to be eaten less frequently, are whole, unrefined grains and pastas. Last of all, and meant to be eaten sparingly—if at all—are refined grains (such as white bread, junk-food cereals, etc.), potatoes, and sweets.

Also in this study, the obese subjects following the slow-carb diet were told to eat non-starchy vegetables (leafy greens, artichoke, asparagus, broccoli, cabbage, mushrooms, onions, peppers, etc.), fruits, beans, nuts, and dairy products. They were instructed to eat carbohydrates with protein, and healthful fats at every meal and snack. They were also instructed to eat until they were full and to snack only when hungry. The other obese people participating in the study were put on a conventional, low-fat/ low-calorie diet. Both groups were asked to exercise regularly and were given lifestyle counseling. Even though the slow-carb dieters were able to eat as much as they wanted and snacked when hungry, they lost as much weight as those told to cut back on fat and calories. Additionally, the slow-carb dieters did better in terms of heart disease risk reduction.[4]

The results showed that after twelve months on the diets, the slow-carb group lost 7.8 percent of their body weight (average sixteen pounds), compared with 6.1 percent (average eleven pounds) in the low-fat group. Likewise, triglyceride levels were down 37 percent in the slow-carb group, compared with 19 percent in the low-fat group (high triglyceride levels are a risk factor in heart disease). Levels of a factor that increases blood clots (plasminogen activator inhibitor) were also decreased by 39 percent in the slow-carb group, but actually increased 33 percent in the low-fat group. Considering that blood clots in the heart arteries are usually the cause of heart attacks, this is a significant improvement.

SLOW-CARB, NOT LOW-CARB

Jennie Brand-Miller, PhD, professor of human nutrition at the University of Sydney, Australia, wrote an editorial that accompanied the slow-carb study in the *American Journal of Clinical*

Nutrition.[5] According to a report on WebMD, Dr. Brand-Miller indicated that the study tells us losing weight on a low-GI diet produces better outcomes in terms of heart health than a conventional weight loss diet. "Even if the amount of weight lost is the same, you are better off on the low-GI diet. So it is a double bonus," she says. Basically, a slow-carb diet is really the opposite of the low-carb diet. With the slow-carb diet, people eat lots of carbohydrates; just selectively. They eat the low-GI versions.

Dr. Brand-Miller's advice for following a slow-carb diet is:

- Aim for heavy-grain breads, sourdough breads, and stone-ground breads.

- Aim for the low-GI breakfast cereals (oats, muesli, bran).

- Aim to eat carbohydrates at every meal.

- Do not avoid any kind of fruit or vegetable except potatoes. Replace white potatoes with sweet potatoes, corn, and other healthy foods.

- Do not be afraid to eat pasta, basmati rice, or couscous.

- Eat lean meat, fish, and chicken.

- Eat lots of legumes (even baked beans).

- Eat nine servings of fruit and vegetables a day.

- Have two to three servings of low-fat dairy a day.

PLANNING YOUR OWN SLOW-CARB DIET

The first step in any diet is to calculate your daily caloric requirements. However, to do this, you need to determine your healthy weight range. Following the steps below will allow you to find out your estimated caloric needs per day and how many calories you need to restrict in order to lose weight.

1. Find your desired weight range using the tables on pages 160 and 161 as guides.[6]

Desirable Weights for Men of Age 25 and Over			
Height	**Weight in pounds according to frame***		
	Small Frame	**Medium Frame**	**Large Frame**
5'1"	112–120	118–129	126–141
5'2"	115–123	121–133	129–144
5'3"	118–126	124–136	132–148
5'4"	121–126	127–139	135–152
5'5"	124–129	130–143	138–156
5'6"	128–137	134–147	142–161
5'7"	132–141	138–152	147–166
5'8"	136–145	142–156	151–170
5'9"	140–150	146–160	155–174
5'10"	144–154	150–165	159–179
5'11"	148–158	154–170	164–184
6'0"	152–162	158–175	168–189
6'1"	156–167	162–180	173–194
6'2"	160–171	167–185	178–199
6'3"	164–175	172–190	182–204

* Fully dressed

2. Multiply this weight (or any number within the weight range) by 15 calories per pound if you are sedentary or 20 calories per pound if you are moderately active. This will give you the number of calories needed per day in order to maintain your current weight.

3. If you want to lose fat, a useful guideline for lowering your calorie intake is to reduce your number of maintainance calories

Desirable Weights for Women of Age 25 and Over

Height	Weight in pounds according to frame*		
	Small Frame	**Medium Frame**	**Large Frame**
4'8"	92–98	96–107	104–119
4'9"	94–101	98–110	106–122
4'10"	96–104	101–113	109–125
4'11"	99–107	104–116	112–128
5'0"	102–110	107–119	115–131
5'1"	105–113	110–122	118–134
5'2"	108–116	113–126	121–138
5'3"	111–119	116–130	125–142
5'4"	114–123	120–135	129–146
5'5"	118–127	124–139	133–150
5'6"	122–131	128–143	137–154
5'7"	126–135	132–147	141–158
5'8"	130–140	136–151	145–163
5'9"	134–144	140–155	149–168
5'10	138–148	144–159	153–173

* Fully dressed

by 500 calories per day. As a guide to minimum calorie intake, the American College of Sports Medicine (ACSM) recommends that calorie levels never drop below 1,200 calories per day for women or 1,800 calories per day for men. Even these calorie levels are quite low. Keep this in mind: if you cut back your calories too much, your metabolism will slow down and you may not lose a pound!

For optimum health and weight control, it is *not* necessary to eat only low-GI foods. However, be sure to choose more of these low-GI foods for your daily diet, or combine one or more low-GI food choices with medium- and high-GI foods in the same meal. As a guideline, the following is a sample menu for a daily diet providing 2,100 calories and incorporating low-GI foods:[7]

Breakfast	1 poached egg *(1 lean protein)*
	2 slices rye toast *(2 unrefined starch)*
	2 ounces Canadian bacon *(2 lean protein)*
	1 cup fresh berries *(1 fruit)*
	1 cup coffee with sweetener
Lunch	4 ounces grilled chicken breast *(4 lean protein)*
	2 cups mixed greens *(2 vegetable)*
	1 cup chopped fresh vegetables *(1 vegetable)*
	2 tablespoons light vinaigrette *(1 sugar)*
	1 cup minestrone soup *(2 unrefined starch)*
Snack	1 banana *(1 fruit)*
	2 tablespoons peanut butter *(1 legume and 1 nut)*
	1 cup low-fat milk *(1 low-fat dairy)*
Dinner	6 ounce broiled salmon filet *(6 lean protein)*
	2 tablespoons fresh lemon juice
	1 cup asparagus spears *(1 vegetable)*
	$1/2$ cup brown rice *(1 unrefined starch)*
	1 cup low-fat milk *(1 low-fat dairy)*
Snack	Handful of almonds *(1 legume and 1 nut)*

You can flavor the foods listed on the menu with herbs and spices. Just watch your intake of condiments such as ketchup, mustard, barbecue sauce, soy sauce, syrup, mayonnaise, salad dressings, sour cream, cream cheese, and oils (especially olive and canola). Moderation is key to all of these ingredients. Calories add up very quickly when using condiments!

The following table will help you make appropriate food choices when planning your own daily menu.

Category	Menu Choices	Recommended Servings Per Day Based on Calorie Intake
Fruits	**Low GI:** Apples, apricots (raw and dried), berries, cherries, grapefruit, grapes, kiwi, lemons, limes, mango, melon, nectarines, papaya, peaches, pineapple, oranges, pears, plums, rhubarb, tomatoes, tomato juice	1,200 calories: 2 1,500 calories: 2 1,800 calories: 2 2,100 calories: 2 2,500 calories: 2 3,000 calories: 3
	Medium GI: Apple juice, bananas, cranberry juice, figs, fruit cocktail (canned in water), grapefruit juice, orange juice, pineapple juice	**1 Serving:** 1 cup fresh; $\frac{1}{2}$ cup juice; $\frac{1}{4}$ cup dried
	High GI: Dates, raisins	
Vegetables	**Low GI:** Artichokes, asparagus, avocado, bok choy, broccoli, Brussels sprouts, cabbage, carrots, cauliflower, celery, chunky salsa, corn, cucumber, eggplant, green beans, green peas, leeks, lettuce (all varieties), marinara sauce, mushrooms, onions, peppers, spinach, tomato soup	1,200 calories: 3 1,500 calories: 4 1,800 calories: 4 2,100 calories: 4 2,500 calories: 4 3,000 calories: 5
	Medium GI: Split pea soup, squash, sweet potatoes, yams, zucchini,	**1 Serving:** 1 cup fresh; $\frac{1}{2}$ cup cooked; $\frac{1}{2}$ cup potatoes; 10 small French fries
	High GI: French fries, potatoes	

Category	Menu Choices	Recommended Servings Per Day Based on Calorie Intake
Lean Protein	**Low GI:** Chicken breast, clams, crab, eggs, fish, lean beef, lean turkey, oysters, pork, scallops, shrimp,	1,200 calories: 7 1,500 calories: 7 1,800 calories: 10 2,100 calories: 11 2,500 calories: 12 3,000 calories: 18 **1 Serving:** 1 ounce lean meat
Low-Fat Dairy	**Low GI:** Cheese, Glucerna diet drink, ice cream (reduced fat and low-calorie), milk, rice milk, soy milk, yogurt (fat free and sugar free **Medium GI:** Chocolate milk, Ensure	1,200 calories: 1 1,500 calories: 1 1,800 calories: 2 2,100 calories: 2 2,500 calories: 2 3,000 calories: 3 **1 Serving:** 1 cup milk; 1 cup low fat yogurt or cottage cheese; 1 inch cube cheese
Nuts and Legumes	**Low GI:** Almonds, baked beans, black beans, black-eyed peas, brazil nuts, butter beans, cashews, chick peas, kidney beans, lentils, macadamia nuts, navy beans, peanut butter, peanuts, pecans, pinto beans, soybeans, walnuts **Medium GI:** Lima beans	1,200 calories: 1 1,500 calories: 1 1,800 calories: 1 2,100 calories: 2 2,500 calories: 2 3,000 calories: 2 **1 Serving:** 1 ounce nuts; $1/2$ cup beans

Category	Menu Choices	Recommended Servings Per Day Based on Calorie Intake
Unrefined Starches	Low GI: All-Bran and Bran Buds cereal, lentil soup, minestrone soup, oat-bran bread, popcorn (plain), pumpernickel bread, rye bread, spelt bread, sugar-free granola, whole wheat bread, whole wheat pasta, whole wheat tortilla, whole wheat waffles,	1,200 calories: 2 1,500 calories: 3 1,800 calories: 4 2,100 calories: 5 2,500 calories: 6 3,000 calories: 6
	Medium GI: Barley, brown rice, corn tortillas, couscous, oatmeal (unsweetend), pasta, pretzels, rice cakes, Chex, Cherrios, Corn Flakes, Grapenuts, Life, Shredded Wheat, and Special K cereals	**1 Serving:** 1 slice bread; 1 small tortilla; $\frac{1}{2}$ cup cereal; $\frac{1}{2}$ cup pasta or rice; 1 cup soup (broth based); 2 tbs hummus; $\frac{1}{2}$ cup oatmeal; $\frac{1}{2}$ bagel; 1 pancake; 1 waffle
	High GI: Bagels, basmati rice, long-grain rice, pancakes, potato chips, stuffing, white rice, Corn Pops, Fruit Loops, Golden Grahams, and Rice Krispies cereals	
Sugars	Low GI: Honey, light salad dressings, Nestle Quik dissolved in low-fat milk	1,200 calories: 1 1,500 calories: 1 1,800 calories: 1
	High GI: Cakes, candy, cookies, donuts, muffins, pancakes, pastries, poptarts, soft drinks, syrup	2,100 calories: 1 2,500 calories: 1 3,000 calories: 2
		1 Serving: 1 small cookie, cake, donut, pancake, poptart, or pastry

Additionally, here are some healthy snack ideas to incorporate into your diet.

- Apple slices with almond butter
- Carrot sticks with hummus
- Celery sticks with peanut butter
- Glass of low-fat chocolate milk
- Handful of pecans
- Hard-boiled egg
- Low-fat yogurt with almonds
- One-half banana with low-fat yogurt
- Peach slices with cottage cheese
- Protein shake made with low-fat milk

Finally, here are some other helpful keys and tips to incorporate into your daily routine.

- Always make sure to drink a full glass of water prior to each meal and snack.

- Decrease the consumption of sugary foods like cookies, candies, and soft drinks.

- If you are looking for lower fat protein sources, try a protein shake (whey or soy protein) made with water or low-fat milk.

- If you consume a high-GI food, be sure to combine it with a low-GI food. A good way to remember to do this is by incorporating some type of protein and fat at every meal and snack (try slices of banana with peanut butter instead of just eating a banana).

- Lean meats usually come from the loin, so choose filet, pork loin, and sirloin instead of ribs and heavily marbled meats.

• Long-term success in any weight management or nutrition improvement program is made easier by keeping a daily food diary. If you keep a log of what you are eating and note serving sizes, time of day you eat your meals and snacks, your mood, how much fluid you drink, your daily overall caloric intake, and your bottom line—your weight—the program becomes an easy part of your daily life.

• Plan your meals ahead of time (especially if you work all day) to make sure that you never go more than four or five hours without eating a meal or healthy snack.

• Select fish that is fresh (preferably not frozen) whenever possible and try to include at least 1 serving of tuna or salmon (high in omega-3 fatty acids) in your diet per week.

• Choose healthy fats/oils (i.e. olive, canola, safflower, or sunflower oils).

• When buying groceries, do most of your shopping where fresh fruits, vegetables, meats, and dairy are found to avoid the temptation of high-GI (processed) foods.

RESOURCES

This appendix will provide you with trustworthy sources, useful dietary supplement brands, organizations, and other types of useful information.

DIETARY SUPPLEMENT BRANDS

The following list provides dietary supplement brands that I recommend based upon my experience in the field. Although these are not the only good dietary supplement brands available, it is my opinion that you can obtain high quality dietary supplements from each of these brands listed.

Arthur Andrew Medical

(480) 385-4791, (800) 448-5015, www.arthurandrew.com
Arthur Andrew Medical (AAM) is a brand sold by healthcare professionals and in vitamin or health food stores. AAM specializes in exotic and clinically effective enzymes and probiotics.

Bronson Laboratories

(800) 235-3200, www.bronsonvitamins.com
Bronson is a direct-to-consumer brand, offering a full line of vitamin, mineral, and specialty products, including products that are specific to diabetics.

Complementary Prescriptions

(888) 401-1105 (patients), (888) 401-0967 (heathcare professionals), www.cpmedical.net/index.aspx
Complementary Prescriptions (CP) is a brand sold by healthcare

professionals. They offer a full line of vitamin, mineral, and innovative specialty products, including products that are specific to diabetics.

Earth Wise

(888) 797-1300, www.earthwisevitamins.com
Earth Wise is a retail brand available in Earth Wise Nutrition Centers, offering a full line of vitamin, mineral, and specialty products.

Futurebiotics

(800) 294-5518, www.futurebiotics.com
Futurebiotics is a retail brand available in many vitamin and health food stores. It offers a full line of specialty formulations, including products that are specific to diabetics.

Jarrow Formulas

(310) 204-6936, www.jarrow.com
Jarrow Formulas (JF) is a retail brand available in many vitamin and health food stores, offering a full line of vitamin, mineral, and specialty products. JF has particularly good probiotic products, including products that are specific to diabetics.

LifeBotanica

(800) 847-6160, www.lifebotanica.com
LifeBotanica is a direct-to-consumer and retail brand available in many vitamin and health food stores. It specializes in herbal detoxification formulations but has plans to extend the line to include an herbal glucose control formula and other herbal products.

Vitamin Research Products

(800) 877-2447, www.vrp.com
Vitamin Research Products (VRP) is a direct-to-consumer and retail brand sold in vitamin and health food stores. VRP offers a full line of vitamin, mineral, and innovative specialty products, including products that are specific to diabetics.

Viva Vitamins

(661) 645-8482, www.vivavitamins.com

Viva Vitamins is a retail brand available in many vitamin/health food stores, offering a full line of vitamin, mineral, and specialty products. These include products that are specific to diabetics.

HEALTHCARE PROFESSIONAL ORGANIZATIONS

If you want to find a healthcare professional to work with regarding nutrition and dietary supplements, contact one or more of the following organizations for a referral to someone in your area.

The American Association of Naturopathic Physicians

(202) 237-8150, (866) 538-2267, www.naturopathic.org

The American Association of Naturopathic Physicians (AANP), which was founded in 1985, is the national professional society representing licensed or licensable naturopathic physicians, all of whom are graduates of four-year, residential graduate programs. Each of the seven schools in North America is either accredited, or is a candidate for accreditation by an agency of the United States Department of Education.

The American Chiropractic Association

(703) 276-8800, www.acatoday.org

The American Chiropractic Association (ACA) is the largest professional association in the world representing doctors of chiropractic. The ACA provides lobbying, public relations, professional and educational opportunities for chiropractic doctors, funds research regarding chiropractic and health issues, and offers leadership for the advancement of the profession.

The American Clinical Board of Nutrition

(540) 635-8844, www.acbn.org

The American Clinical Board of Nutrition (ACBN), which was founded in 1986, is a professional certification organization that works to establish education, examination, experience, and ethics requirements for certification.

The American Herbalists Guild

(203) 272-6731, www.americanherbalistsguild.com

The American Herbalists Guild was founded in 1989 as a non-profit, educational organization to represent the goals and voices of herbalists specializing in the medicinal use of plants. Its primary goal is to promote a high level of professionalism and education in the study and practice of therapeutic herbalism.

The National Association of Nutrition Professionals

(800) 342-8037, www.nanp.org

The National Association of Nutrition Professionals (NANP) is a non-profit business league of nutrition professionals that was founded in 1985. It represents holistically trained nutrition professionals. Its mission is to enhance the integrity of the holistic nutrition profession through self-governance, educational standards, a rigorous code of ethics, and professional registration of holistic nutritionists.

The Certification Board for Nutrition Specialists

(727) 446-6086, www.cbns.org

Founded in 1993, the Certification Board for Nutrition Specialists aims to help meet the growing demand for knowledgeable, responsible, professional nutritionists.

LOCATING A PERSONAL CHEF

As mentioned in Chapter 9, a personal chef can be an extremely useful tool for losing weight and eating healthier, especially for people who don't have time to prepare and cook nutritious meals.

United States Personal Chef Association

(800) 995-2138, www.uspca.com

To find your own qualified personal chef, I recommend that you visit the website for the United States Personal Chef Association and click on the link that reads "Hire a Personal Chef." On two occasions I have spoken at the conference for this organization, and both times I have found that it is a professional group with sensitivity to special dietary needs.

SELF-EDUCATION ABOUT DIETARY SUPPLEMENTS

The following list includes reputable sources, should you want to learn about dietary supplements.

The American Botanical Council

(512) 926-4900, (800) 373-7105, http://abc.herbalgram.org

Established in 1988, the American Botanical Council (ABC) is the leading independent, nonprofit, international member-based organization that provides education using science-based and traditional information to promote the responsible use of herbal medicine. ABC serves the public, researchers, educators, health-care professionals, industry, and media.

The Council for Responsible Nutrition

(202) 204-7700, www.crnusa.org

Founded in 1973, the Council for Responsible Nutrition (CRN) is the leading trade association representing dietary supplement manufacturers and ingredient suppliers. CRN companies produce a large portion of the dietary supplements marketed both in the United States and globally.

The Dietary Supplement Information Bureau

(202) 204-4723, www.supplementinfo.org

The Dietary Supplement Information Bureau (DSIB) was founded in 2001 to promote the responsible use of vitamins, minerals, herbs, and specialty supplements. DSIB is committed to ensuring that consumers, the media, healthcare professionals, and policy-makers have the complete facts about dietary supplements.

Huntington College of Health Sciences

(865) 524-8079, (800) 290-4226, www.hchs.edu

Huntington College of Health Sciences offers more than a conventional undergraduate or graduate education. Its accredited distance learning degrees and diploma programs include the breadth of responsible complementary and alternative medicine viewpoints, providing students with a well-rounded and integrative approach to nutrition and dietary supplement science. The college also offers full-length courses in nutritrion and dietary supplement science.

The Linus Pauling Institute's Micronutrient Information Center

(541) 737-5075, http://lpi.oregonstate.edu/infocenter/

The Linus Pauling Institute's Micronutrient Information Center is a source for scientifically accurate information regarding the roles of vitamins, minerals, other nutrients, dietary phytochemicals, and some foods in preventing disease and promoting health. All of the nutrients and phytochemicals included in the Micronutrient Information Center may be obtained from the diet, but many are also available as dietary supplements.

Natural Products Association

(202) 223-0101, www.npainfo.org/

The Natural Products Association (NPA) was founded in 1936 and is the nation's largest and oldest non-profit organization dedicated to the natural products industry. NPA represents more than 10,000 retailers, manufacturers, wholesalers, and distributors of natural products.

NSF International

(800) 673-8010, www.nsf.org/

NSF International, The Public Health and Safety Company, is a not-for-profit, non-governmental organization. It is the world leader in standards development, product certification, education, and risk-management for public health and safety.

APPENDIX C

COMPLEMENTARY THERAPIES

The following list explains each of the complementary therapies in discussed in this book.

ACUPOINT MASSAGE. A massage technique based on the principles of acupuncture. It is characterized by pressing and rubbing on acupuncture meridians, acupoints, muscles, and skin areas with different parts of the palms and fingers and varying degrees of force.[1]

ACUPUNCTURE. Acupuncture involves inserting and manipulating fine filiform (thread-like) needles into specific meridian points on the body. Acupuncture has been extensively studied and has been shown to be effective in treating some conditions, particularly certain forms of pain.[2]

According to the National Center for Complementary and Alternative Medicine, traditional Chinese medicine (TCM) is a system of healing that dates back to 200 B.C. in written form.[3] TCM sees the body as a delicate balance between yin and yang, two opposing and inseparable forces. The cold, slow, or passive principle is Yin. The hot, excited, or active principle is yang. TCM assumes that health is achieved by maintaining a balanced state in the body. Disease, therefore, is due to an internal imbalance of yin and yang. This imbalance leads to blockage in the flow vital energy known as of qi (pronounced "chee") and of blood along pathways known as meridians.

The concept that sickness and disease arise from vital energy imbalances has led to a series of approaches that are taken to rectify the flow of qi. Acupuncture is the most well known of these approaches.

ACUPRESSURE. A traditional Chinese medicine (TCM) technique derived from acupuncture. In acupressure, physical pressure is applied to acupuncture points by the hand, elbow, or with various devices.

BIOFEEDBACK. A technique in which various monitoring devices are used to help a person learn to voluntarily alter body functions that are normally involuntary, such as brain activity, blood pressure, muscle tension, or heart rate. Biofeedback can be administered in a number of ways. An electromyogram (EMG) uses electrodes or other sensors to measure muscle tension. By showing people when their muscles are tensed, it can help them learn to relax these muscles, possibly alleviating such conditions as backaches, headaches, and neck pain, which are sometimes associated with muscle tension. It can also be helpful for medical conditions that are worsened by stress, such as asthma. In temperature biofeedback, sensors are attached to the person's fingers or feet to measure skin temperature. A low skin temperature reading may indicate stress, so such a reading can serve as a prompt to begin relaxation techniques. This type of biofeedback may be useful in easing conditions related to circulation, including migraines and peripheral vascular disease. Regular biofeedback can be given by an appropriately trained technician, or you may be trained to administer biofeedback to yourself. Contact the Biofeedback Association of North America for more information by going to http://biofeedbackassociation.com. Temperature biofeedback generally requires a technician.

EXERCISE. If you think that exercise is not really a complementary therapy, you are right. Nevertheless, given the frequency (or lack thereof) with which many people integrate exercise into their lifestyles, exercise might as well be an alternative, non-mainstream health practice. A recent government report says seven in ten adults do not exercise regularly and nearly four out of ten are not physically active at all; and these figures did not change from

1997 to 2001.[4] Furthermore, exercise as a complementary treatment for conditions of the cardiovascular and pulmonary systems, mood disorders, and the disabilities associated with aging can in many cases reverse or improve disease conditions.[5]

Although you may already know this, let us take this opportunity to identify the two major types of exercise: aerobic and resistance training. Aerobic training consists of those exercises that utilize large muscle groups (such as those found in the legs) at a low level of intensity, for an extended period of time (twenty minutes or longer). Examples of aerobic exercise include jogging, brisk walking, bicycling, or the treadmill. Aerobic training is best for promoting cardiovascular fitness and burning body fat. On the contrary, resistance training consists of placing stress upon different muscle groups, which helps to improve their tone and increase their size. Examples of resistance training include weight lifting, dynamic tension, and calisthenics.

Before starting an exercise program, you should get approval from your doctor since exercise can exacerbate certain physical problems, as well as have an effect on blood sugar levels.

HYPNOSIS. A mental state induced by a procedure known as a hypnotic induction. Hypnotic induction is commonly composed of a series of preliminary instructions and suggestions. Hypnotic suggestions may be delivered by a hypnotist in the presence of the subject, or they may be self-administered. The use of hypnotism for therapeutic purposes is referred to as "hypnotherapy." During hypnosis, the subject is in a wakeful state of focused attention and heightened suggestibility, with diminished peripheral awareness.

MAGNET THERAPY. A complementary and alternative medicine practice involving the use of magnetic fields or electromagnetic radiation. Magnetic fields currently play an important role in Western medicine, as is the case with magnetic resonance imaging (MRI). Magnet therapy is sometimes used by patients on their own, or it can be administered by healthcare providers. Magnet therapy may be applied to the whole body or only to areas affected by illness. The magnetic fields produced by static magnets are different from electromagnetic radiation and are likely to have different effects on the body. Typically, magnets are worn on specific parts of the body for extended periods of time (for example, two weeks).[6] Magnet therapy was originally considered pseudoscience, primarily due to inconsistent research findings.[7-9] However, more systematic research has confirmed that strong static magnetic fields from permanent magnets are able to constrict and dilate the walls of capillary blood vessels.[10,11] This reduces inflammation and increases blood circulation, respectively.[12] Static magnet therapy has potentially effective applications in relief of pain and swelling after a sports injury and blunt trauma, as well as wound healing after surgery.[13,14]

MEDITATION. A mental discipline by which one attempts to get beyond the reflexive "thinking" mind into a deeper state of relaxation or awareness. Meditation often involves turning attention to a single point of reference. It is a component of many religions, and has been practiced for many, many years. Some religions even include meditation as part of their spiritual practices.

Different meditative disciplines encompass a wide range of spiritual or psychophysical practices that may emphasize different goals, from achievement of a higher state of consciousness; to greater focus, creativity, or self-awareness; or simply a more relaxed and peaceful frame of mind. From the point of view of psychology and physiology, meditation can induce an altered state of consciousness, and its goals in that context have been stated as achieving spiritual enlightenment, transforming attitudes, and better cardiovascular health.

MOXIBUSTION. A traditional Chinese medicine technique that involves burning the herb mugwort to facilitate healing. The method preferred by modern practitioners is referred to as "indirect moxibustion." There are different ways in which this can be done. Two of the most common methods include a practitioner either lighting one end of a moxa stick (about the shape and size of a cigar) and holding it close to the area being treated for several minutes until the area turns red, or inserting an acupuncture needle into an acupoint, wrapping moxa around the tip of the needle, and then igniting it to generate heat to the point and the surrounding area. As with most forms of traditional Chinese medicine, the purpose of moxibustion is to strengthen the blood, stimulate the flow of qi, and maintain general health.[15]

OXYHYDROMASSAGE. The consumption of oxygen-rich mineral water and hydromassage (applying massage techniques through the water) are methods used to increase oxygen levels in the human body, independent of breathing it in through your lungs. The combination of the two methods is called oxyhydromassage.[16]

RELAXATION TRAINING. A program that consists of any method, process, procedure, or activity that helps an individual relax, attain a state of increased calmness, or otherwise reduce levels of anxiety, stress, or tension. Various techniques are used by individuals to improve their state of relaxation. Some of the methods are performed alone, and some require the help of another person, often a trained professional. Some involve movement, while others focus on stillness. Biofeedback and deep breathing are examples of two relaxation techniques.

TAI CHI. Tai chi was originally developed in China as a form of self-defense. It is a graceful form of exercise that has existed for centuries. Practiced regularly, tai chi can help you reduce stress and enjoy other health benefits. Tai chi is a noncompetitive, self-paced system of gentle physical exercise and stretching. To do tai chi, you perform a series of postures or movements in a slow, graceful manner. Each posture flows into the next, without a pause in between.[17]

TRANSCENDENTAL MEDITATION (TM).   A meditation technique introduced in 1958 by Maharishi Mahesh Yogi (1917–2008). In TM, the subject mentally recites a special mantra (sacred sound or phrase). Concentration on the repeated utterances decreases mental activity, and as a result the subject is expected to reach a higher state of consciousness. Taught in a standardized seven-step course by certified teachers, the technique is practiced for fifteen to twenty minutes twice per day, while sitting comfortably with closed eyes.

YOGA.   Yoga is a healing system of theory and practice, and there are different ways of practicing it. The word is associated with meditative practices in Hinduism, Buddhism, and Jainism. It is a combination of breathing exercises, physical postures, and meditation aimed at training the consciousness to promote control of the body and mind. It has been practiced for centuries. There are a number of major branches of yoga in Hindu philosophy, with the most well known in Western culture being Hatha Yoga. Compared to other branches of yoga, which are often performed while seated, Hatha yoga uses full body "postures" that are now in popular usage with many modern variations that many people associate with the word "yoga" today.[18] Many yoga schools and classes are readily available throughout the United States and in many other parts of the world. Whichever one you attend, make sure you are taught by an accredited yoga instructor.

APPENDIX D

BODY MASS INDEX

Body Mass Index (BMI) provides a reliable indicator of body fat by taking height and weight into consideration. It is used to screen for weight categories that may lead to health problems.

To calculate your BMI, use one of the formulas below or go to the National Heart Lung and Blood Institute's website for an online calculator (www.nhlbisupport.com/bmi/).

Calculate Your Body Mass Index Using BMI Formulas

Body Mass Index (BMI) is a number calculated from a person's weight and height. To see where you fall on the BMI scale, put your height and weight into the equation below.

$$\frac{\text{Weight (in pounds)} \times 703}{\text{Height (in inches)}^2} = \text{BMI}$$

Or, if you prefer to use kilograms and meters instead of pounds and inches, you can use the following equation.

$$\frac{\text{Weight (in kilograms)}}{\text{Height (in meters)}^2} = \text{BMI}$$

What Does Your BMI Mean? If it's:

- Below 18.5: You are considered underweight.
- Between 18.5 and 24.9: You are considered normal weight.
- Between 25 and 29.9: You are considered overweight.
- Above 30: You are considered obese.

REFERENCES

Chapter 1

1. Rolfes, S.R.; Pinna, K.; Whitney, E. *Understanding Normal and Clinical Nutrition, 7th Edition.* Belmont, CA: Thomson Wadsworth, 2006.

2. Rolfes, S.R.; Pinna, K.; Whitney, E. *Understanding Normal and Clinical Nutrition, 7th Edition.* Belmont, CA: Thomson Wadsworth, 2006.

3. National Institute of Diabetes and Digestive and Kidney Diseases. National Diabetes Statistics, 2007 fact sheet. Bethesda, MD: U.S. Department of Health and Human Services. National Institutes of Health, 2008.

4. National Institute of Diabetes and Digestive and Kidney Diseases. National Diabetes Statistics, 2007 fact sheet. Bethesda, MD: U.S. Department of Health and Human Services. National Institutes of Health, 2008.

5. National Institute of Diabetes and Digestive and Kidney Diseases. National Diabetes Statistics, 2007 fact sheet. Bethesda, MD: U.S. Department of Health and Human Services. National Institutes of Health, 2008.

6. The U.S. Department of Health and Human Services National Diabetes Education Program. If you have diabetes . . . know your blood sugar numbers! NIH Publication No. 98-4350, Revised July 2005.

7. The U.S. Department of Health and Human Services National Diabetes Education Program. If you have diabetes . . . know your blood sugar numbers! NIH Publication No. 98-4350, Revised July 2005.

Chapter 2

1. Kulkarni, K. "Diets do not fail: the success of medical nutrition therapy in patients with diabetes." *Endocr Pract.* 2006; 12 Suppl 1: 121–123.

2. Mendoza, D. Revised International Table of Glycemic Index (GI) and Glycemic Load (GL) Values. 2008. Last modified: December 16, 2008. Retrieved September 8, 2009. www.mendosa.com/gilists.htm

3. Thomas, D.; Elliott, E.J. "Low glycaemic index, or low glycaemic load, diets for diabetes mellitus." *Cochrane Database Syst Rev.* 2009; 1: CD006296.

4. Riccardi, G.; Rivellese, A.A.; Giacco, R. "Role of glycemic index and glycemic load in the healthy state, in prediabetes, and in diabetes." *Am J Clin Nutr.* 2008; 87(1): 269S—274S.

5. Sartorelli, D.S.; Cardoso, M.A. "Association between dietary carbohydrates and type 2 diabetes mellitus: epidemiological evidence." *Arq Bras Endocrinol Metabol.* 2006; 50(3): 415–426.

6. Lapinleimu, H.; Viikari, J.; Jokinen, E.; et al. "Prospective randomised trial in 1062 infants of diet low in saturated fat and cholesterol." *Lancet.* 1995; 345(8,948): 471–476.

7. Francisco Fuentes; José López-Miranda; Elias Sánchez; Francisco Sánchez; José Paez; Elier Paz-Rojas; Carmen Marín; Purificación Gómez; José Jimenez-Perepérez; José M. Ordovás; Francisco Pérez-Jiménez. "Mediterranean and Low-Fat Diets Improve Endothelial Function in Hypercholesterolemic Men." *Annals of Internal Medicine.* 2001; 134(12): 1,115–1,119.

8. Hu, F.B.; Stampfer, M.J.; Manson, J.E.; et al. "Dietary fat intake and the risk of coronary heart disease in women." *N Engl J Med.* 1997; 337(21): 1,491–1,499.

9. Lapinleimu, H.; Viikari, J.; Jokinen, E.; et al. "Prospective randomised trial in 1062 infants of diet low in saturated fat and cholesterol." *Lancet.* 1995; 345(8,948): 471–476.

10. Lovejoy, J.C. "The influence of dietary fat on insulin resistance." *Current Diabetes Reports.* 2002; 2(5): 435–440.

11. Fedor, D.; Kelley, D.S. "Prevention of insulin resistance by n-3 polyunsaturated fatty acids." *Curr Opin Clin Nutr Metab Care.* 2009; 12(2): 138–146.

12. Vassiliou, E.K.; Gonzalez, A.; Garcia, C.; Tadros, J.H.; Chakraborty, G.; Toney, J.H. "Oleic acid and peanut oil high in oleic acid reverse the inhibitory effect of insulin production of the inflammatory cytokine TNF-alpha both in vitro and in vivo systems." *Lipids Health Dis.* 2009; 8: 25.

13. Mozaffarian, D.; Katan, M.B.; Ascherio, A.; Stampfer, M.J.; Willett, W.C. "Trans fatty acids and cardiovascular disease." *N Engl J Med.* 2006; 354(15): 1,601–1,613.

14. Emily Sonestedt; Ulrika Ericson; Bo Gullberg; Kerstin Skog; Håkan Olsson; Elisabet Wirfält. "Do both heterocyclic amines and omega-6 polyunsaturated fatty acids contribute to the incidence of breast cancer in postmenopausal women of the Malmö diet and cancer cohort?" *The International Journal of Cancer.* 2008; 123(7): 1,637–1,643.

15. Yong, Q.; Chen; et al. "Modulation of prostate cancer genetic risk by

omega-3 and omega-6 fatty acids." *Journal of Clinical Investigation.* 2007; 117(7): 1,866.

16. Strychar, I.; Cohn, J.S.; Renier, G.; Rivard, M.; Aris-Jilwan, N.; Beauregard, H.; Meltzer, S.; Belanger, A.; Dumas, R.; Ishac, A.; Radwan, F.; Yale, J.F. "Effects of a Higher-Carbohydrate/Lower-Fat Diet Versus a Lower-Carbohydrate/Higher-Fat-Monounsaturated Diet on Postmeal Triglyceride Concentrations and other Cardiovascular Risk Factors in Type 1 Diabetes." *Diabetes Care.* 2009.

17. Walker, C.; Reamy, B.V. "Diets for cardiovascular disease prevention: what is the evidence?" *Am Fam Physician.* 2009; 79(7): 571–578.

18. Mente, A.; de Koning, L.; Shannon, H.S.; Anand, S.S. "A systematic review of the evidence supporting a causal link between dietary factors and coronary heart disease." *Arch Intern Med.* 2009; 169(7): 659–669.

19. Shai, I.; Schwarzfuchs, D.; Henkin, Y.; et al. "Weight loss with a low-carbohydrate, Mediterranean, or low-fat diet." *N Engl J Med.* 2008; 359(3): 229–241.

20. Agatston, A. *The South Beach Diet.* St. Martins Press, 2003.

21. Aude, Y.W.; Agatston, A.S.; Lopez-Jimenez, F.; Lieberman, E.H., Marie Almon; Hansen, M.; Rojas, G.; Lamas, G.A.; Hennekens, C.H. "The national cholesterol education program diet vs a diet lower in carbohydrates and higher in protein and monounsaturated fat: a randomized trial." *Arch Intern Med.* 2004; 164(19): 2,141–2,146.

22. Link, L.B.; Jacobson, J.S. "Factors affecting adherence to a raw vegan diet." *Complement Ther Clin Pract.* 2008; 14(1): 53–59.

23. Douglass, J.M. "Raw diet and insulin requirements." *Ann Intern Med.* 1975; 82(1): 61–62.

24. Fontana, L.; Meyer, T.E.; Klein, S.; Holloszy, J.O. "Long-term low-calorie low-protein vegan diet and endurance exercise are associated with low cardiometabolic risk." *Rejuvenation Res.* 2007; 10(2): 225–234.

25. Koebnick, C.; Garcia, A.L.; Dagnelie, P.C.; Strassner, C.; Lindemans, J.; Katz, N.; Leitzmann, C.; Hoffmann, I. "Long-term consumption of a raw food diet is associated with favorable serum LDL cholesterol and triglycerides but also with elevated plasma homocysteine and low serum HDL cholesterol in humans." *J Nutr.* 2005; 135(10): 2,372–2,378.

26. Donaldson, M.S. "Metabolic vitamin B12 status on a mostly raw vegan diet with follow-up using tablets, nutritional yeast, or probiotic supplements." *Ann Nutr Metab.* 2000; 44(5–6): 229–234.

27. Key, T.J.; Thorogood, M.; Appleby, P.N.; Burr, M.L. "Dietary habits and

mortality in 11,000 vegetarians and health conscious people: results of a 17 year-follow up." *BMJ*. 1996; 313(7,060): 775–779.

28. Link, L.B.; Hussaini, N.S.; Jacobson, J.S. "Change in quality of life and immune markers after a stay at a raw vegan institute: a pilot study." *Complement Ther Med*. 2008; 16(3): 124–130.

29. Krebs-Smith, S.M.; Kris-Etherton, P. "How does MyPyramid compare to other population-based recommendations for controlling chronic disease?" *J Am Diet Assoc*. 2007; 107(5): 830–837.

30. Krebs-Smith, S.M.; Kris-Etherton, P. "How does MyPyramid compare to other population-based recommendations for controlling chronic disease?" *J Am Diet Assoc*. 2007; 107(5): 830–837.

31. Atkins, R.C. *Dr. Atkins' New Diet Revolution*. New York: Quill, 2002. 47–55.

32. Brehm, B.J.; Seeley, R.J.; Daniels, S.R.; et al. "A Randomized Trial Comparing a Very Low Carbohydrate Diet and a Calorie-Restricted Low Fat Diet on Body Weight and Cardiovascular Risk Factors in Healthy Women." *Journal of Clinical Endocrinology and Metabolism*. 2003; 88(4): 1,617–1,623.

33. Foster, G.D.; Wyatt, H.R.; Hill, J.O.; et al. "A Randomized Trial of a Low-Carbohydrate Diet for Obesity." *New England Journal of Medicine*. 2003; 348(21): 2,082–2,090.

34. Organic Food Standards and Labels: The Facts. The Organic National Food Program. May 25, 2005. www.ams.usda.gov/AMSv1.0/nop.

35. Kristensen, E.S. "Food safety in an organic perspective." 14th IFOAM Congress. Victoria, Canada; August 22nd 2002. Accessed May 25, 2005. http://orgprints.org/19/03/Kristensen_IFOAM_2002.ppt.

36. Holmboe-Ottesen, G. "Better health with ecologic food?" *Tidsskrift for den Norske laegeforening*. 2004; 124(11): 1,529–1,531.

37. Kristensen, E.S. "Food safety in an organic perspective." 14th IFOAM Congress. Victoria, Canada; August 22nd 2002. Accessed May 25, 2005. http://orgprints.org/19/03/Kristensen_IFOAM_2002.ppt.

38. Magkos, F.; Arvaniti, F.; Zampelas, A. "Organic food: nutritious food or food for thought? A review of the evidence." *International Journal of Food Sciences and Nutrition*. 2003; 54(5): 357–371.

39. Holmboe-Ottesen, G. "Better health with ecologic food?" *Tidsskrift for den Norske laegeforening*. 2004; 124(11): 1,529–1,531.

40. Magkos, F.; Arvaniti, F.; Zampelas, A. "Organic food: nutritious food or food for thought? A review of the evidence." *International Journal of Food Sciences and Nutrition*. 2003; 54(5): 357–371.

41. Holmboe-Ottesen, G. "Better health with ecologic food?" *Tidsskrift for den Norske laegeforening*. 2004; 124(11): 1,529–1,531.

Chapter 3

1. Kodentsova, V.M.; Pustograev, N.N.; Vrzhesinskaia, O.A.; Kharitonchik, L.A.; Pereverzeva, O.G.; Iakushina, L.M.; Trofimenko, L.S.; Spirichev, V.B. "Comparison of metabolism of water-soluble vitamins in healthy children and in children with insulin-dependent diabetes mellitus depending upon the level of vitamins in the diet." *Vopr Med Khim*. 1996; 42(2): 153–158.

2. Report Card on the Quality of Americans' Diets. Nutrition Insights, INSIGHT 28. USDA Center for Nutrition Policy and Promotion. December 2002.

3. Johnson-Spruill, I.; Hammond, P.; Davis, B.; McGee, Z.; Louden, D. "Health of Gullah families in South Carolina with type 2 diabetes: diabetes self-management analysis from project SuGar." *Diabetes Educ*. 2009; 35(1): 117–123.

4. Rovner, A.J.; Nansel, T.R. "Are children with type 1 diabetes consuming a healthful diet?: a review of the current evidence and strategies for dietary change." *Diabetes Educ*. 2009; 35(1): 97–107.

5. Gerrior, S.; Bente, L. "Nutrient Content of the U.S. Food Supply, 1909-94." U.S. Department of Agriculture, Center for Nutrition Policy and Promotion. Home Economics Report No. 53., 1997.

6. Alpaslan, M.; Gunduz, H. "The effects of growing conditions on oil content, fatty acid composition and tocopherol content of some sunflower varieties produced in Turkey." *Die Nahrung*. 2000; 44(6): 434–437.

7. USDA National Nutrient Database for Standard Reference, Release 15. USDA Nutrient Data Laboratory. December 11, 2002.

8. Barta, D.J.; Tibbitts, T.W.; Barta, D.J. "Calcium localization and tipburn development in lettuce leaves during early enlargement." *Journal of the American Society for Horticultural Science*. 2000; 125(3): 294–298.

9 Hou, T.Z.; Mooneyham, R.E. "Applied studies of plant meridian system: I. The effect of agri-wave technology on yield and quality of tomato." *American Journal of Chinese Medicine*. 1999; 27(1): 1–10.

10. McKeehen, J.D.; Smart, D.J.; Mackowiak, C.L.; et al. "Effect of CO_2 levels on nutrient content of lettuce and radish. Advances in space research." *The Official Journal of the Committee on Space Research*. 1996; 18(4–5): 85–92.

11. Kubota, J.; Allaway, W.H. "Geographic distribution of trace element problems. "Micronutrients in Agriculture." Proceedings of Symposium

held at Muscle Shoals, Alabama; Madison, WI. Soil Science Society of America; 1972: 525–554.

12. "Composition of Foods: Raw, Processed, Prepared." USDA National Nutrient Database for Standard Reference, Release 15. December 2002.

13. Williams, P.G. "Vitamin retention in cook/chill and cook/hot-hold hospital food-services." *J Am Diet Assoc*. 1996; 96: 490–498.

14. Fletcher, R.H.; Fairfield, K.M. "Vitamins for Chronic Disease Prevention in Adults." *JAMA*. 2002; 287(23): 3,127–3,129.

15. National Center for Health Statistics. "Use of dietary supplements in the United States, 1988-94." Vital and Health Statistics from the Centers for Disease Control and Prevention, Series 11, No. 244, June 1999.

16. Nutrition Business Journal. "NBJ's annual overview of the nutrition industry VI." *Nutrition Business Journal*. 2001; VI (5–6): 1–7, 17–18.

17. Kaufman, D.W.; Kelly, J.P.; Rosenberg, L.; Anderson, T.E.; Mitchell, A.A. "Recent patterns of medication use in the ambulatory adult population of the United States: The Slone Survey." *J Am Med Assn*. 2002; 287: 337–344.

18. Miggiano, G.A.D.; Gagliardi, L. "Diabetes and diet revisited." *La Clinica terapeutica*. 2006; 157(5): 443–455.

19. Sanchez-Alvarez, J.E.; Perez-Tamajon, L.; Hernandez, D.; Alvarez-Gonzalez, A.; Delgado, P.; Lorenzo, V. "Efficacy and safety of two vitamin supplement regimens on homocysteine levels in hmodialysis patients. Prospective, randomized clinical trial." *Nefrologia*. 2005; 25(3): 288–296.

20. Spano, M. "Choosing a multivitamin." *Diabetes self-management*. 2007; 24(3): 46, 48–50, 52, 54.

21. Ahmed, N.; Thornalley, P.J. "Advanced glycation endproducts: what is their relevance to diabetic complications?" *Diabetes Obes Metab*. 2007; 9(3): 233–245.

22. Wautier, J.L.; Schmidt, A.M. "Protein Glycation: A Firm Link to Endothelial Cell Dysfunction." *Circ Res*. 2004; 95: 233–238.

23. Ahmed, N.; Thornalley, P.J. "Advanced glycation endproducts: what is their relevance to diabetic complications?" *Diabetes Obes Metab*. 2007; 9(3): 233–245.

24. Ceriello, A. "New Insights on Oxidative Stress and Diabetic Complications May Lead to a 'Causal' Antioxidant Therapy." *Diabetes Care*. 2003; 26: 1,589–1,596.

25. Wright Jr., E.; Scism-Bacon, L.; Glass, L.C. "Oxidative stress in type 2 diabetes: the role of fasting and postprandial glycaemia." *Int J Clin Pract*. 2006; 60(3): 308–314.

26. Giugliano, D.; Ceriello, A.; Paolisso, G. "Oxidative stress and diabetic vascular complications." *Diabetes Care.* 1996; 19(3): 257–267.

27. Chertow, B. "Advances in diabetes for the millennium: vitamins and oxidant stress in diabetes and its complications." *Med Gen Med.* 2004; 6(3 Suppl): 4.

28. Sauberlich, H.E. "Implications of nutritional status on human biochemistry, physiology, and health." *Clin Biochem.* 1984; 17(2): 132–142.

29. Bjorkegren, K.; Svardsudd. "Elevated serum levels of methylmalonic acid and homocysteine in elderly people. A population-based intervention study." *J Intern Med.* 1999; 246(3): 317–324.

30. Rasmussen, K.; Moller, J.; Lyngbak, M. "Within-person variation of plasma homocysteine and effects of posture and tourniquet application." *Clin Chem.* 1999; 45(10): 1,850–1,855.

31. Kunz, K.; Petitjean, P.; Lisri, M.; et al. « Cardiovascular morbidity and endothelial dysfunction in chronic haemodialysis patients: Is homocyst(e)ine the missing link?" *Nephrol Dial Transplant.* 1999; 14(8): 1,934–1,942.

32. Alpert, M.A. "Homocysteine, atherosclerosis, and thrombosis." *South Med J.* 1999; 92(9): 858–865.

33. Bellamy, M.F.; McDowell, I.F.; Ramsey, M.W.; et al. "Oral folate enhances endothelial function in hyperhomocysteinaemic subjects." *Eur J Clin Invest.* 1999; 29(8): 659–662.

34. Woodside, J.V.; Young, I.S.; Yarnell, J.W.G.; et al. "Antioxidants, but not B-group vitamins increase the resistance to low-density lipoprotein to oxidation: a randomised, factorial design, placebo-controlled trial." *Atherosclerosis.* 1999; 144(2): 419–427.

35. Bronstrup, A.; Hages, M.; Pietrzik, K. "Lowering of homocysteine concentrations in elderly men and women." *Int J Vitam Nutr Res.* 1999; 69(3): 187–193.

36. Suliman, M.E.; Divino Filho, J.C.; Barany, P.; et al. "Effects of high-dose folic acid and pyridoxine on plasma and erythrocyte sulfur amino acids in hemodialysis patients." *J Am Soc Nephrol.* 1999; 10(6): 1,287–1,296.

37. Mansoor, M.A.; Kristensen, O.; Hervig, T.; et al. "Plasma total homocysteine response to oral doses of folic acid and pyridoxine hydrochloride (vitamin B6) in healthy individuals. Oral doses of vitamin B6 reduce concentration of serum folate." *Scand J Clin Lab Invest.* 1999; 59(2): 139–146.

38. Abahusain, M.A.; Wright, J.; Dickerson, J.W.; de Vol, E.B. "Retinol, alpha-tocopherol and carotenoids in diabetes." *Eur J Clin Nutr.* 1999; 53(8): 630–635.

39. Polidori, M.C.; Mecocci, P.; Stahl, W.; et al. "Plasma levels of lipophilic

antioxidants in very old patients with type-2 diabetes." *Diabetes Metab Res Rev.* 2000; 16: 15–19.

40. Siemianowicz, K.; Gminski, J.; Telega, A.; Wójcik, A.; Posielezna, B.; Grabowska-Bochenek, R.; Francuz, T. "Blood antioxidant parameters in patients with diabetic retinopathy." *Int J Mol Med.* 2004; 14(3): 433–437.

41. Pittas, A.G.; Lau, J.; Hu, F.; Dawson-Hughes, B. "The Role of Vitamin D and Calcium in type 2 diabetes. A systematic Review and Meta-Analysis." *J Clin Endocrinol Metab.* 2007; 92(6): 2,017–2,029.

42. Herbert, V. "Vitamin B-12." *Present Knowledge in Nutrition. 7th ed.* Washington, D.C.: ILSI Press, 1996; 191–205.

43. Davies, S.; Howard, J.M.; Hunnisett, A.; et al. "Age-related decreases in chromium levels in 51,665 hair, sweat, and serum samples from 40,872 patients—implications for the prevention of cardiovascular disease and type II diabetes." *Metabolism.* 1997; 46: 469–473.

44. Morris, B.W.; Kemp, G.J.; Hardisty, C.A. "Plasma chromium and chromium excretion in diabetes." *Clin Chem.* 1985; 31: 334–335.

45. Anderson, R.A.; Cheng, N.; Bryden, N.A.; et al. "Elevated intakes of supplemental chromium improve glucose and insulin variables in individuals with type 2 diabetes." *Diabetes.* 1997; 46: 1,786–1,791.

46. Rabinovitz, H.; Friedensohn, A.; Leibovitz, A.; et al. "Effect of chromium supplementation on blood glucose and lipid levels in type 2 diabetes mellitus elderly patients." *Int J Vitam Nutr Res.* 2004; 74: 178–182.

47. Martin, J.; Wang, Z.Q.; Zhang, X.H.; et al. "Chromium picolinate supplementation attenuates body weight gain and increases insulin sensitivity in subjects with type 2 diabetes." *Diabetes Care.* 2006; 29: 1,826–1,832.

48. Ascherio, A.; Willett, W.C.; Rimm, E.B.; Giovannucci, E.L.; Stampfer, M.J. "Dietary iron intake and risk of coronary disease among men." *Circulation.* 1994; 89(3): 969–974.

49. Klipstein-Grobusch, K.; Grobbee, D.E.; den Breeijen, J.H.; Boeing, H.; Hofman, A.; Witteman, J.C. "Dietary iron and risk of myocardial infarction in the Rotterdam Study." *Am J Epidemiol.* 1999; 149(5): 421–428.

50. De Valk, B.; Marx, J.J. "Iron, atherosclerosis, and ischemic heart disease." *Arch Intern Med.* 1999; 159(14): 1,542–1,548.

51. Food and Nutrition Board, Institute of Medicine. Iron. "Dietary reference intakes for vitamin A, vitamin K, boron, chromium, copper, iodine, iron, manganese, molybdenum, nickel, silicon, vanadium, and zinc." Washington D.C.: National Academy Press; 2001: 290–393.

52. Barbagallo, M.; Dominguez, L.J.; Resnick, L.M. "Magnesium metabo-

lism in hypertension and type 2 diabetes mellitus." *Am J Ther.* 2007; 14(4): 375–385.

53. Meyer, K.A.; Kushi, L.H.; Jacobs, D.R.; et al. "Carbohydrates, dietary fiber, and incident type 2 diabetes in older women." *Am J Clin Nutr.* 2000; 71: 921–930.

54. Song, Y.; Manson, J.E.; Buring, J.E.; Liu, S. "Dietary magnesium intake in relation to plasma insulin levels and risk of type 2 diabetes in women." *Diabetes Care.* 2004; 27: 59–65.

55. Fung, T.T.; Manson, J.E.; Solomon, C.G.; et al. "The association between magnesium intake and fasting insulin concentration in healthy middle-aged women." *J Am Coll Nutr.* 2003; 22: 533–538.

56. Lopez-Ridaura, R.; Willett, W.C.; Rimm, E.B.; et al. "Magnesium intake and risk of type 2 diabetes in men and women." *Diabetes Care.* 2004; 27: 134–140.

57. Larsson, S.C.; Wolk, A. "Magnesium intake and risk of type-2 diabetes: a meta-analysis." *J Intern Med.* 2007; 262: 208–214.

58. Johnson, P.E.; Lykken, G.I. "Manganese and calcium absorption and balance in young women fed diets with varying amounts of manganese and calcium." *J Trace Elem Exp Med.* 1991; 4: 19–35.

59. El-Yazigi, A.; Hannan, N.; Raines, D.A. "Urinary excretion of chromium, copper, and manganese in diabetes mellitus and associated disorders." *Diabetes Res.* 1991; 18(3):129–134.

60. Davis, R.E.; Calder, J.S.; Curnow, D.H. "Serum pyridoxal and folate concentrations in diabetics." *Pathology.* 1976; 8: 151–156.

61. McCann, V.J.; Davis, R.E. "Serum pyridoxal concentrations in patients with diabetic neuropathy." *Aust N Z J Med.* 1978; 8: 259–261.

62. Chetyrkin, S.V.; Mathis, M.E.; Ham, A.J.; Hachey, D.L.; Hudson, B.G.; Voziyan, P.A. "Propagation of protein glycation damage involves modification of tryptophan residues via reactive oxygen species: inhibition by pyridoxamine." *Free Radic Biol Med.* 2008; 44(7): 1,276–1,285.

63. Nobécourt, E.; Zeng, J.; Davies, M.J.; Brown, B.E.; Yadav, S.; Barter, P.J.; Rye, K.A. "Effects of cross-link breakers, glycation inhibitors and insulin sensitizers on HDL function and the non-enzymatic glycation of apolipoprotein A-I." *Diabetologia.* 2008; 51(6): 1,008–1,017.

64. Voziyan, P.A.; Hudson, B.G. "Pyridoxamine: the many virtues of a maillard reaction inhibitor." *Ann N Y Acad Sci.* 2005; 1,043: 807–816.

65. Voziyan, P.A.; Hudson, B.G. "Pyridoxamine as a multifunctional phar-

maceutical: targeting pathogenic glycation and oxidative damage." *Cell Mol Life Sci.* 2005; 62(15): 1,671–1,681.

66. Will, J.C.; Byers, T. "Does diabetes mellitus increase the requirement for vitamin C?" *Nutr Rev.* 1996; 54: 193–202.

67. Peerapatdit, T.; Patchanans, N.; Likidlilid, A.; Poldee, S.; Sri-ratanasathavorn, C. "Plasma lipid peroxidation and antioxidiant nutrients in type 2 diabetic patients." *J Med Assoc Thai.* 2006; 89 Suppl 5: 147–155.

68. Siemianowicz, K.; Gminski, J.; Telega, A.; Wójcik, A.; Posielezna, B.; Grabowska-Bochenek, R.; Francuz, T. "Blood antioxidant parameters in patients with diabetic retinopathy." *Int J Mol Med.* 2004; 14(3): 433–437.

69. Chertow, B. "Advances in diabetes for the millennium: vitamins and oxidant stress in diabetes and its complications." *Med Gen Med.* 2004; 6(3 Suppl): 4.

70. Davie, S.J.; Gould, B.J.; Yudkin, J.S. "Effect of vitamin C on glycosylation of proteins." *Diabetes.* 1992; 41: 167–173.

71. Will, J.C.; Byers, T. "Does diabetes mellitus increase the requirement for vitamin C?" *Nutr Rev.* 1996; 54: 193–202.

72. McAuliffe, A.V.; Brooks, B.A.; Fisher, E.J.; et al. "Administration of ascorbic acid and an aldose reductase inhibitor (tolrestat) in diabetes: effect on urinary albumin excretion." *Nephron.* 1998; 80: 277–284.

73. Millen, A.E.; Klein, R.; Folsom, A.R.; et al. "Relation between intake of vitamins C and E and risk of diabetic retinopathy in the Atherosclerosis Risk in Communities Study." *Am J Clin Nutr.* 2004; 79: 865–873.

74. Osganian, S.K.; Stampfer, M.J.; Rimm, E.; et al. "Vitamin C and risk of coronary heart disease in women." *J Am Coll Cardiol.* 2003; 42(2): 246–252.

75. Chiu, K.C.; Chu, A.; Go, V.L.W.; Saad, M.F. "Hypovitaminosis D is associated with insulin resistance and β-cell dysfunction." *Am J Clin Nutr.* 2004; 79: 820–825.

76. Schwalfenberg, G. "Vitamin D and diabetes: Improvement of glycemic control with vitamin D3 repletion." *Can Fam Physician.* 2008; 54: 864–866.

77. Borissova, A.M.; Tankova, T.; Kirilov, G.; Dakovska, L.; Kovacheva, R. "The effect of vitamin D3 on insulin secretion and peripheral insulin sensitivity in type 2 diabetic patients." *Int J Clin Pract.* 2003; 57(4): 258–261.

78. Orwoll, E.; Riddle, M.; Prince, M. :Effects of vitamin D on insulin and glucagon secretion in non-insulin-dependent diabetes mellitus." *Am J Clin Nutr.* 1994; 59(5): 1,083–1,087.

79. Inomata, S.; Kadowaki, S.; Yamatani, T.; Fukase, M.; Fujita, T." Effect of

1 alpha (OH)-vitamin D3 on insulin secretion in diabetes mellitus." *Bone Miner.* 1986; 1(3): 187–192.

80. Peerapatdit, T.; Patchanans, N.; Likidlilid, A.; Poldee ,S,. Sriratanasathavorn, C. "Plasma lipid peroxidation and antioxidant nutrients in type 2 diabetic patients." *J Med Assoc Thai.* 2006; 89 Suppl 5: S147–S155.

81. Polidori, M.C.; Mecocci, P.; Stahl, W.; et al. "Plasma levels of lipophilic antioxidants in very old patients with type 2 diabetes." *Diabetes Metab Res Rev.* 2000; 16: 15–19.

82. Siemianowicz, K.; Gminski, J.; Telega, A.; Wójcik, A.; Posielezna, B.; Grabowska-Bochenek, R.; Francuz, T. "Blood antioxidant parameters in patients with diabetic retinopathy." *Int J Mol Med.* 2004; 14(3): 433–437.

83. Jain, S.K.; McVie, R.; Jaramillo, J.J.; et al. "Effect of modest vitamin E supplementation on blood glycated hemoglobin and triglyceride levels and red cell indices in type I diabetic patients." *J Am Coll Nutr.* 1996; 15: 458–461.

84. Jain, S.K.; McVie, R.; Jaramillo, J.J.; et al. "Effect of modest vitamin E supplementation on blood glycated hemoglobin and triglyceride levels and red cell indices in type I diabetic patients." *J Am Coll Nutr.* 1996; 15: 458–461.

85. Ceriello, A.; Giugliano, D.; Quatraro, A.; et al. "Vitamin E reduction of protein glycosylation in diabetes. New prospect for prevention of diabetic complications?" *Diabetes Care.* 1991; 14: 68–72.

86. Duntas, L.; Kemmer, T.P.; Vorberg, B.; Scherbaum, W. "Administration of d-alpha-tocopherol in patients with insulin-dependent diabetes mellitus." *Curr Ther Res.* 1996; 57: 682–690.

87. Brody, T. *Nutritional Biochemistry. 2nd ed.* San Diego: Academic Press, 1999.

88. Shearer, M.J. "The roles of vitamins D and K in bone health and osteoporosis prevention." *Proc Nutr Soc.* 1997; 56(3): 915–937.

89. Shearer, M.J. "Vitamin K." *Lancet.* 1995; 345(8,944): 229–234.

90. Roe, D.A. "Drug and nutrient interactions in the elderly diabetic." *Drug Nutr Interact.* 1988; 5(4): 195–203.

91. Whitney, E.; Cataldo, C.; Rolfes, S. *Understanding Normal and Clinical Nutrition, Fifth Edition.* Belmont, California: West/Wadsworth; 1998, 434.

92. Whitney, E.; Cataldo, C.; Rolfes, S. *Understanding Normal and Clinical Nutrition, Fifth Edition.* Belmont, California: West/Wadsworth; 1998, 419.

93. Yung, S.; Mayersohn, M.; Robinson, J.B. "Ascorbic acid absorption in humans: a comparison among several dosage forms." *Journal of pharmaceutical sciences.* 1982; 71(3): 282–285.

94. Bland, J. *Bioflavonoids.* New Canaan, Connecticut: Keats Publishing; 1984, 18–20.

95. Machlin, L.J.; Brin, M. "Bioequivalence of RRR-alpha- tocopheryl acetate and all-rac-alpha-tocopheryl acetate." *Am J Clin Nutr.* 1981; 34(8): 1,633–1,636.

Chapter 4

1. Packer, L.; Witt, E.H.; Tritschler, H.J. "Alpha-Lipoic acid as a biological antioxidant." *Free Rad Biol Med.* 1995; 19: 227–250.

2. Kagan, V.; Khan, S.; Swanson, C.; et al. "Antioxidant action of thioctic acid and dihydrolipoic acid." *Free Radic Biol Med.* 1990; 9S: 15.

3. Jacob, S.; Ruus, P.; Hermann, R.; et al. "Oral administration of RAC-alpha-lipoic acid modulates insulin sensitivity in patients with type-2 diabetes mellitus: a placebo-controlled, pilot trial." *Free Rad Biol Med.* 1999; 27: 309–314.

4. Konrad, T.; Vicini, P.; Kusterer, K.; et al. "Alpha-lipoic acid treatment decreases serum lactate and pyruvate concentrations and improves glucose effectiveness in lean and obese patients with Type 2 diabetes." *Diabetes Care.* 1999; 22: 280–287.

5. Jacob, S.; Henriksen, E.J.; Tritschler, H.J.; et al. "Improvement of insulin-stimulated glucose-disposal in type 2 diabetes after repeated parenteral administration of thioctic acid." *Exp Clin Endocrinol Diabet.* 1996; 104: 284–288.

6. Jacob, S.; Henriksen, E.J.; Schiemann, A.L.; et al. "Enhancement of glucose disposal in patients with type 2 diabetes by alpha-lipoic acid." *Arzneimittelforschung.* 1995; 45: 872–874.

7. Vincent, H.K.; Bourguignon, C.M.; Vincent, K.R.; Taylor, A.G. "Effects of alpha-lipoic acid supplementation in peripheral arterial disease: a pilot study." *J Alt Complement Med.* 2007; 13: 577–584.

8. Konrad, T.; Vicini, P.; Kusterer, K.; et al. "Alpha-lipoic acid treatment decreases serum lactate and pyruvate concentrations and improves glucose effectiveness in lean and obese patients with Type 2 diabetes." *Diabetes Care.* 1999; 22: 280–287.

9. Albarracin, C.; Fuqua, B.; Evans, J.L.; Goldfine, I.D. "Chromium picolinate and biotin combination improves glucose metabolism in treated, uncontrolled overweight to obese patients with type 2 diabetes." *Diabetes Metab Res Rev.* 2008; 24: 41–51.

10. Albarracin, C.; Fuqua, B.; Evans, J.L.; Goldfine, I.D. "Chromium picolinate and biotin combination improves glucose metabolism in treated,

uncontrolled overweight to obese patients with type 2 diabetes." *Diabetes Metab Res Rev.* 2008; 24: 41–51.

11. Baez-Saldana, A.; Zendejas-Ruiz, I.; Revilla-Monsalve, C.; et al. "Effects of biotin on pyruvate carboxylase, acetyl-CoA carboxylase, propionyl-CoA carboxylase, and markers for glucose and lipid homeostasis in type 2 diabetic patients and nondiabetic subjects." *Am J Clin Nutr.* 2004; 79: 238–243.

12. Davies, S.; Howard, J.M.; Hunnisett, A.; et al. "Age-related decreases in chromium levels in 51,665 hair, sweat, and serum samples from 40,872 patients – implications for the prevention of cardiovascular disease and type II diabetes." *Metabolism.* 1997; 46: 469–473.

13. Morris, B.W.; Kemp, G.J.; Hardisty, C.A. "Plasma chromium and chromium excretion in diabetes." *Clin Chem.* 1985; 31: 334–335.

14. Anderson, R.A.; Cheng, N.; Bryden, N.A.; et al. "Elevated intakes of supplemental chromium improve glucose and insulin variables in individuals with type 2 diabetes." *Diabetes.* 1997; 46: 1,786–1,791.

15. Rabinovitz, H.; Friedensohn, A.; Leibovitz, A.; et al. "Effect of chromium supplementation on blood glucose and lipid levels in type 2 diabetes mellitus elderly patients." *Int J Vitam Nutr Res.* 2004; 74: 178–182.

16. Martin, J.; Wang, Z.Q.; Zhang, X.H.; et al. "Chromium picolinate supplementation attenuates body weight gain and increases insulin sensitivity in subjects with type 2 diabetes." *Diabetes Care.* 2006; 29: 1,826–1,832.

17. Martin, J.; Wang, Z.Q.; Zhang, X.H.; et al. "Chromium picolinate supplementation attenuates body weight gain and increases insulin sensitivity in subjects with type 2 diabetes." *Diabetes Care.* 2006; 29: 1,826–1,832.

18. Anderson, R.A.; Cheng, N.; Bryden, N.A.; et al. "Elevated intakes of supplemental chromium improve glucose and insulin variables in individuals with type 2 diabetes." *Diabetes.* 1997; 46: 1,786–1,791.

19. Lee, N.A.; Reasner, C.A. "Beneficial effect of chromium supplementation on serum triglyceride levels in NIDDM." *Diabetes Care.* 1994; 17: 1,449–1,452.

20. Anderson, R.A.; Cheng, N.; Bryden, N.A.; et al. "Elevated intakes of supplemental chromium improve glucose and insulin variables in individuals with type 2 diabetes." *Diabetes.* 1997; 46: 1,786–1,791.

21. Fox, G.N.; Sabovic, Z. "Chromium picolinate supplementation for diabetes mellitus." *J Fam Pract.* 1998; 46: 83–86.

22. Ravina, A.; Slezak, L.; Mirsky, N.; et al. "Reversal of corticosteroid-

induced diabetes mellitus with supplemental chromium." *Diabet Med.* 1999; 16: 164–167.

23. Anderson, R.A. "Chromium in the prevention and control of diabetes." *Diabetes Metab.* 2000; 26: 22–27.

24. Fox, G.N.; Sabovic, Z. "Chromium picolinate supplementation for diabetes mellitus." *J Fam Pract.* 1998; 46(1) :83–86.

25. Mertz, W. "Interaction of chromium with insulin: a progress report." *Nutr Rev.* 1998; 56: 174–177.

26. John-Kalarickal, J.; Pearlman, G.; Carlson, H.E. "New medications which decrease levothyroxine absorption." *Thyroid.* 2007; 17: 763–765.

27. Baker, W.L.; Gutierrez-Williams, G.; White, C.M.; et al. "Effect of cinnamon on glucose control and lipid parameters." *Diabetes Care.* 2008; 31: 41–43.

28. Mang, B.; Wolters, M.; Schmitt, B.; Kelb, K.; Lichtinghagen, R.; Stichtenoth, D.O.; Hahn, A. "Effects of a cinnamon extract on plasma glucose, HbA, and serum lipids in diabetes mellitus type 2." *European Journal of Clinical Investigation.* 2006; 36: 340–344

29. Ziegenfguss, T.N.; Hofheins, J.E.; Mendel, R.W.; Landis, J.; Anderson, R.A. "Effects of a Water-Soluble Cinnamon Extract on Body Composition and Features of the Metabolic Syndrome in Pre-Diabetic Men and Women." *Journal of the International Society of Sports Nutrition.* 2006; 3(2): 45–53.

30. Baskaran, K.; Kizar-Ahamath, B.; Shanmugasundaram, M.R.; Shanmugasundaram, E.R.B. "Antidiabetic effect of leaf extract from Gymnema sylvestre in non-insulin-dependent diabetes mellitus patients." *J Ethnopharmacol.* 1990; 30: 295–300.

31. Shanmugasundaram, E.R.; Rajeswari, G.; Baskaran, K.; et al. "Use of Gymnema sylvestre leaf extract in the control of blood glucose in insulin-dependent diabetes mellitus." *J Ethnopharmacol.* 1990; 30: 281–294.

32. Huseini, H.F.; Larijani, B.; Heshmat, R.; et al. "The efficacy of Silybum marianum (L.) Gaertn. (silymarin) in the treatment of type II diabetes: a randomized, double-blind, placebo-controlled, clinical trial." *Phytother Res.* 2006; 20; 1,036–1,039.

33. Huseini, H.F.; Larijani, B.; Heshmat, R.; et al. "The efficacy of Silybum marianum (L.) Gaertn. (silymarin) in the treatment of type II diabetes: a randomized, double-blind, placebo-controlled, clinical trial." *Phytother Res.* 2006; 20; 1,036–1,039.

34. Sotaniemi, E.A.; Haapakoski, E.; Rautio, A. "Ginseng therapy in non-insulin dependent diabetic patients." *Diabetes Care*. 1995; 18: 1,373–1,375.

35. Vuksan, V.; Sung, M.K.; Sievenpiper, J.L.; Stavro, P.M.; Jenkins, A.L.; Di Buono, M.; Lee, K.S.; Leiter, L.A.; Nam, K.Y.; Arnason, J.T.; Choi, M.; Naeem, A. "Korean red ginseng (Panax ginseng) improves glucose and insulin regulation in well-controlled, type 2 diabetes: results of a randomized, double-blind, placebo-controlled study of efficacy and safety." *Nutr Metab Cardiovasc Dis*. 2008; 18(1): 46–56.

36. Sotaniemi, E.A.; Haapakoski, E.; Rautio, A. "Ginseng therapy in non-insulin dependent diabetic patients." *Diabetes Care*. 1995; 18: 1,373–1,375.

37. Shin, H.R.; Kim, J.Y.; Yun, T.K.; et al. "The cancer-preventive potential of Panax ginseng: a review of human and experimental evidence." *Cancer Causes Control*. 2000; 11: 565–576.

38. Liu, X.; Zhou, H.J.; Rohdewald, P. "French maritime pine bark extract pycnogenol dose-dependently lowers glucose in type 2 diabetic patients (letter)." *Diabetes Care*. 2004; 27: 839.

39. Liu, X.; Wei, J.; Tan, F.; et al. "Antidiabetic effect of Pycnogenol French maritime pine bark extract in patients with diabetes type II." *Life Sci*. 2004; 75: 2,505–2,513.

40. Gill, J.M.; Cooper, A.R. "Physical activity and prevention of type 2 diabetes mellitus." *Sports Med*. 2008; 38(10): 807–824.

41. O'Gorman, D.J.; Krook, A. "Exercise and the treatment of diabetes and obesity." *Endocrinol Metab Clin North Am*. 2008; 37(4): 887–903.

42. Gordon, B.A.; Benson, A.C.; Bird, S.R.; Fraser, S.F. "Resistance training improves metabolic health in type 2 diabetes: a systematic review." *Diabetes Res Clin Pract*. 2009; 83(2): 157–175.

43. Loimaala, A.; Groundstroem, K.; Rinne, M.; Nenonen, A.; Huhtala, H.; Parkkari, J.; Vuori, I. "Effect of long-term endurance and strength training on metabolic control and arterial elasticity in patients with type 2 diabetes mellitus." *Am J Cardiol*. 2009; 103(7): 972–977.

44. Tucker, P.S.; Fisher-Wellman, K.; Bloomer, R.J. "Can exercise minimize postprandial oxidative stress in patients with type 2 diabetes?" *Curr Diabetes Rev*. 2008; 4(4): 309–319.

45. Chipkin, S.R.; Klugh, S.A.; Chasan-Taber, L. "Exercise and diabetes." *Cardiol Clin*.

46. Watters, K.H. "A holistic approach to meeting students' needs: using hypnotherapy techniques to assist students in managing their health." *J School Nurs*. 1998; 14: 44–48.

47. Ratner, H.; Gross, L.; Casas, J.; Castells, S. "A hypnotherapeutic approach to the improvement of compliance in adolescent diabetics." *Am J Clin Hypnosis.* 1990; 32: 154–159.

48. Ratner, H.; Gross, L.; Casas, J.; Castells, S. "A hypnotherapeutic approach to the improvement of compliance in adolescent diabetics." *Am J Clin Hypnosis.* 1990; 32: 154–159.

49. McEwen, B.S. "Protective and damaging effects of stress mediation." *N Engl J Med.* 1998; 329: 1,246–1,253.

50. Ornish, D.; Brown, S.E.; Scherwitz, L.V.; Billings, J.H.; Armstrong, W.T.; Ports, T.A.; McLanahan, S.M.; Kirkeelde, R.L.; Brand, R.J.; Gould, K.L.. "Can lifestyle changes reverse coronary heart disease?" *Lancet.* 1990; 336: 129–133.

51. Curtis, J.D.; Deter, R.A.; Schindler, J.V.; Zirkel, J. *Teaching Stress Management & Relaxation Skills: An Instructor's Guide.* La Crosse, WI: Coulee Press; 1985.

52. Guthrie, D.; Moeller, T.; Guthrie, R. "Biofeedback and its application to the stabilization of diabetes." *Am J Clin Biofeedback.* 1987; 2: 82–87.

53. Rice, B.I. "Mind-Body Interventions." *Diabetes Spectrum.* 2001; 14(4): 213–217.

54. Bailey, B.K.; McGrady, A.V.; Good, M. "Management of a patient with insulin- dependent diabetes mellitus learning biofeedback-assisted relaxation." *Diabetes Educ.* 1990; 16: 201–204.

55. McGrady, A.; Gerstenmaier, L. "Effect of biofeedback-assisted relaxation training on blood glucose levels in a type I insulin dependent diabetic: a case report." *J Behav Ther Exper Psychiatr.* 990; 21: 69–75.

56. Cox, D.J.; Taylor, A.G.; Holley-Wilcox, P.; Pohl, S.L.; Guthrow, E. "The relationship between psychological stress and insulin-dependent diabetic blood glucose control: preliminary investigations." *Health Psychol.* 1984; 3: 63–75.

57. Guthrie, D.; Moeller, T.; Guthrie, R. "Biofeedback and its application to the stabilization of diabetes." *Am J Clin Biofeedback.* 1987; 2: 82–87.

58. McGrady, A.; Bailey, B.K.; Good, M.P. "Controlled study of biofeedback-assisted relaxation in type I diabetes." *Diabetes Care.* 1991; 5: 360–365.

59. Jablon, S.L.; Naliboff, B.D.; Gilmore, S.L.; Rosenthal, M.J. "Effects of relaxation training on glucose tolerance and diabetic control in type II diabetes." *Appl Psychophysiol Biofeedback.* 1997; 22: 155–169.

60. Lane, J.D.; McCaskill, C.C.; Ross, S.L.; Feinglos, M.N.; Surwit, R.S.

"Relaxation training for NIDDM: predicting who may benefit." *Diabetes Care.* 1993; 16: 1,087–1,094.

61. Rice, B.I. "Mind-Body Interventions." *Diabetes Spectrum.* 2001; 14(4): 213–217.

62. Alexander, G.K.; Taylor, A.G.; Innes, K.E.; Kulbok, P.; Selfe, T.K. "Contextualizing the effects of yoga therapy on diabetes management: a review of the social determinants of physical activity." *Fam Community Health.* 2008; 31(3): 228–239.

63. Gimbel, M.A. "Yoga, meditation, and imagery: clinical applications." *Nurse Pract Forum.* 1998; 9: 243–255.

64. Jain, S.C.; Uppal, A.; Bhatnagar, S.O.; Talukdar, B. "A study of response pattern of non-insulin dependent diabetics to yoga therapy." *Diabetes Res Clin Pract.* 1993; 19: 69–74.

65. Innes, K.E.; Vincent, H.K. "The influence of yoga-based programs on risk profiles in adults with type 2 diabetes mellitus: a systematic review." *Evid Based Complement Alternat Med.* 2007; 4(4): 469–486.

66. Rice, B.I. "Mind-Body Interventions." *Diabetes Spectrum.* 2001; 14(4): 213–217.

Chapter 5

1. Diabetic Neuropathies: The Nerve Damage of Diabetes. NIH Publication No. 08–3,185. Bethesda, MD: National Diabetes Information Clearinghouse, National Institute of Diabetes and Digestive and Kidney Diseases, National Institutes of Health. February 2008. Retrieved October 3, 2008. http://diabetes.niddk.nih.gov/dm/pubs/neuropathies/.

2. Diabetic Neuropathies: The Nerve Damage of Diabetes. NIH Publication No. 08–3,185. Bethesda, MD: National Diabetes Information Clearinghouse, National Institute of Diabetes and Digestive and Kidney Diseases, National Institutes of Health. February 2008. Retrieved October 3, 2008. http://diabetes.niddk.nih.gov/dm/pubs/neuropathies/.

3. Sima, A.A.F.; Calvani, M.; Mehra, M.; et al. "Acetyl-L-carnitine improves pain, nerve regeneration, and vibratory perception in patients with chronic diabetic neuropathy: An analysis of two randomized, placebo-controlled trials." *Diabetes Care.* 2005; 28: 89–94.

4. Onofrj, M.; Fulgente, T.; Melchionda, D.; et al. "L-acetylcarnitine as a new therapeutic approach for peripheral neuropathies with pain." *Int J Clin Pharmacol Res.* 1995; 15: 9–15.

5. De Grandis, D.; Minardi, C. "Acetyl-L-carnitine (levacecarnine) in the

treatment of diabetic neuropathy. A long-term, randomised, double-blind, placebo-controlled study." *Drugs R D.* 2002; 3: 223–231.

6. Quatraro, A.; Roca, P.; Donzella, C.; et al. "Acetyl-L-carnitine for symptomatic diabetic neuropathy." *Diabetologia.* 1995; 38: 123.

7. Sima, A.A.F.; Calvani, M.; Mehra, M.; et al. "Acetyl-L-carnitine improves pain, nerve regeneration, and vibratory perception in patients with chronic diabetic neuropathy: An analysis of two randomized, placebo-controlled trials." *Diabetes Care.* 2005; 28: 89–94.

8. Martinez, E.; Domingo, P.; Roca-Cusachs, A. "Potentiation of acenocoumarol action by L-carnitine." *J Intern Med.* 1993; 233: 94.

9. Bachmann, H.U.; Hoffmann, A. "Interaction of food supplement L-carnitine with oral anticoagulant acenocoumarol." *Swiss Med Wkly.* 2004; 134: 385.

10. Kagan, V.; Khan, S.; Swanson, C.; et al. "Antioxidant action of thiotic acid and dihydrolipoic acid." *Free Radic Biol Med.* 1990; 9S: 15.

11. Ziegler, D.; Hanefeld, M.; Ruhnau, K.; et al. "Treatment of symptomatic diabetic polyneuropathy with the antioxidant alpha-lipoic acid: A 7-month, multicenter, randomized, controlled trial (ALADIN III Study)." *Diabetes Care.* 1999; 22: 1,296–1,301.

12. Reljanovic, M.; Reichel, G.; Rett, K.; et al. "Treatment of diabetic polyneuropathy with the antioxidant thioctic acid (alpha-lipoic acid): A 2-year, multicenter, randomized, double-blind, placebo-controlled trial (ALADIN II). Alpha Lipoic Acid in Diabetic Neuropathy." *Free Radic Res.* 1999; 31: 171–177.

13. Ziegler, D.; Hanefeld, M.; Ruhnau, K.J.; et al. "Treatment of symptomatic diabetic peripheral neuropathy with the antioxidant alpha-lipoic acid: A 3-week, multicenter, randomized, controlled trial (ALADIN Study)." *Diabetologia.* 1995; 38: 1,425–1,433.

14. Ruhnau, K.J.; Meissner, H.P.; Finn, J.R.; et al. "Effects of 3-week oral treatment with the antioxidant thioctic acid (alpha-lipoic acid) in symptomatic diabetic polyneuropathy." *Diabet Med.* 1999; 16: 1,040–1,043.

15. Ametov, A.S.; Barinov, A.; Dyck, P.J.; et al. "The sensory symptoms of diabetic polyneuropathy are improved with alpha-lipoic acid." *Diabetes Care.* 2003; 26: 770–776.

16. Ziegler, D.; Nowak, H.; Kemplert, P.; et al. "Treatment of symptomatic diabetic polyneuropathy with the antioxidant alpha-lipoic acid: A meta-analysis." *Diabet Med.* 2004; 21: 114–121.

17. Negrisanu, G.; Rosu, M.; Bolte, B.; Lefter, D.; Dabelea, D. "Effects of 3-

month treatment with the antioxidant alpha-lipoic acid in diabetic peripheral neuropathy." *Rom J Intern Med.* 1999; 37: 297–306.

18. Zeigler, D.; Schatz, H.; Conrad, F.; Gries, F.A.; Ulrich, H.; Reichel, G. "Effects of treatment with the antioxidant alpha-lipoic acid on cardiac autonomic neuropathy in NIDDM patients. A 4-month randomized controlled multicenter trial (DEKAN Study)." *Deutsche Kardiale Autonome Neuropathie. Diabetes Care.* 1997; 20: 369–373.

19. Tankova, T.; Cherninkova, S.; Koev, D. "Treatment for diabetic mononeuropathy with alpha-lipoic acid." *Int J Clin Pract.* 2005; 59: 645–650.

20. Konrad, T.; Vicini, P.; Kusterer, K.; et al. "Alpha-lipoic acid treatment decreases serum lactate and pyruvate concentrations and improves glucose effectiveness in lean and obese patients with Type 2 diabetes." *Diabetes Care.* 1999; 22: 280–287.

21. Jacob, S.; Henriksen, E.J.; Tritschler, H.J.; et al. "Improvement of insulin-stimulated glucose-disposal in type 2 diabetes after repeated parenteral administration of thioctic acid." *Exp Clin Endocrinol Diabet.* 1996; 104: 284–288.

22. Jacob, S.; Henriksen, E.J.; Schiemann, A.L.; et al. "Enhancement of glucose disposal in patients with type 2 diabetes by alpha-lipoic acid." *Arzneimittelforschung.* 1995; 45: 872–874.

23. Jacob, S.; Ruus, P.; Hermann, R.; et al. "Oral administration of RAC-alpha-lipoic acid modulates insulin sensitivity in patients with type -2 diabetes mellitus: a placebo-controlled, pilot trial." *Free Rad Biol Med.* 1999; 27: 309–314.

24. Konrad, T.; Vicini, P.; Kusterer, K.; et al. "Alpha-lipoic acid treatment decreases serum lactate and pyruvate concentrations and improves glucose effectiveness in lean and obese patients with Type 2 diabetes." *Diabetes Care.* 1999; 22: 280–287.

25. Sachse, G.; Willms, B. "Efficacy of thioctic acid in the therapy of peripheral diabetic neuropathy." *Hormone Metab Res.* Suppl 1,980; 9: 105–107.

26. Vincent, H.K.; Bourguignon, C.M.; Vincent, K.R.; Taylor, A.G. "Effects of alpha-lipoic acid supplementation in peripheral arterial disease: a pilot study." *J Alt Complement Med.* 2007; 13: 577–584.

27. Haupt, E.; Ledermann, H.; Kopcke, W. "Benfotiamine in the treatment of diabetic polyneuropathy – a three-week randomized, controlled pilot study (BEDIP study)." *Int J Clin Pharmacol Ther.* 2005; 43: 71–77.

28. Winkler, G.; Pál, B.; Nagybéganyi, E.; Ory, I.; Porochnavec, M.; Kempler, P. "Effectiveness of different benfotiamine dosage regimens in the treatment of painful diabetic neuropathy." *Arzneimittelforschung.* 1999; 49(3): 220–224.

29. Head, K.A. "Peripheral neuropathy: pathogenic mechanisms and alternative therapies." *Altern Med Rev.* 2006; 11(4): 294–329.

30. Jamal, G.A. "The use of gamma linolenic acid in the prevention and treatment of diabetic neuropathy." *Diabet Med.* 1994; 11: 145–149.

31. Horrobin, D.F. "The use of gamma-linolenic acid in diabetic neuropathy." *Agents Actions.* Suppl 1992; 37: 120–144.

32. Jamal, G.A.; Carmichael, H. "The effect of gamma-linolenic acid on human diabetic peripheral neuropathy: a double-blind placebo-controlled trial." *Diabet Med.* 1990; 7: 319–323.

33. Keen, H.; Payan, J.; Allawi, J.; et al. "Treatment of diabetic neuropathy with gamma-linolenic acid. The gamma-Linolenic Acid Multicenter Trial Group." *Diabetes Care.* 1993; 16: 8–15.

34. Keen, H.; Payan, J.; Allawi, J.; et al. "Treatment of diabetic neuropathy with gamma-linolenic acid. The gamma-Linolenic Acid Multicenter Trial Group." *Diabetes Care.* 1993; 16: 8–15.

35. Leventhal, L.J.; Boyce, E.G.; Zurier, R.B. "Treatment of rheumatoid arthritis with gammalinolenic acid." *Ann Intern Med.* 1993; 119: 867–873.

36. Zurier, R.B.; Rossetti, R.G.; Jacobson, E.W.; et al. "Gamma-linolenic acid treatment of rheumatoid arthritis. A randomized, placebo-controlled trial." *Arthritis Rheum.* 1996; 39: 1,808–1,817.

37. Keen, H.; Payan, J.; Allawi, J.; et al. "Treatment of diabetic neuropathy with gamma-linolenic acid. The gamma-Linolenic Acid Multicenter Trial Group. *Diabetes Care.* 1993; 16: 8–15.

38. Guivernau, M.; Meza, N.; Barja, P.; Roman, O. "Clinical and experimental study on the long-term effect of dietary gamma-linolenic acid on plasma lipids, platelet aggregation, thromboxane formation, and prostacyclin production." *Prostaglandins Leukot Essent Fatty Acids.* 1994; 51: 311–316.

39. Schalin-Karrila, M.; Mattila, L.; Jansen, C.T.; et al. "Evening primrose oil in the treatment of atopic eczema: effect on clinical status, plasma phospholipid fatty acids and circulating blood prostaglandins." *Br J Dermatol.* 1987; 117: 11–19.

40. Mansel, R.E.; Pye, J.K.; Hughes, L.E. "Effects of essential fatty acids on cyclical mastalgia and noncyclical breast disorders. In Omega-6 Essential Fatty Acids: Pathophysiology and Roles in Clinical Medicine, ed." DF Horrobin. New York: Alan R Liss, 1990, 557–566.

41. Puolakka, J.; Makarainen, L.; Viinikka, L.; Ylikorkola, O. "Biochemical and clinical effects of treating the premenstrual syndrome with prostaglandin synthesis precursors." *J Reprod Med.* 1985; 30: 149–153.

42. Pullman-Mooar, S.; Laposata, M.; Lem, D.; et al. "Alteration of the cellular fatty acid profile and the production of eicosanoids in human monocytes by gamma-linolenic acid." *Arthritis Rheum.* 1990; 33: 1,526–1,533.

43. Yaqub, B.A.; Siddique, A.; Sulimani, R. "Effects of methylcobalamin on diabetic neuropathy." *Clin Neurol Neurosurg.* 1992; 94: 105–111.

44. Yoshioka, K.; Tanaka, K. "Effect of methylcobalamin on diabetic autonomic neuropathy as assessed by power spectral analysis of heart rate variations." *Horm Metab Res.* 1995; 27: 43–44.

45. Ide, H.; Fujiya, S.; Asanuma, Y.; et al. "Clinical usefulness of intrathecal injection of methylcobalamin in patients with diabetic neuropathy." *Clin Ther.* 1987; 9: 183–192.

46. Tatro, D.S. "Drug Interactions Facts. Facts and Comparisons Inc." St. Louis, MO; 1999.

47. Brunelli, B.; Gorson, K.C. "The use of complementary and alternative medicines by patients with peripheral neuropathy." *J Neurol Sci.* 2004; 15; 218(1–2): 59–66.

48. Zhao, M.Y.; Chang, H. "Effect of medicated bath plus acupoint massage on limbs in treating 42 patients with diabetic peripheral neuropathy." *Zhongguo Zhong Xi Yi Jie He Za Zhi.* 2006; 26(11): 1,026–1,028.

49. Mayo Clinic. "Acupuncture." www.mayoclinic.com/health/acupuncture/SA00086.

50. Jiang, H.; Shi, K.; Li, X.; et al. "Clinical study on the wrist-ankle acupuncture treatment for 30 cases of diabetic peripheral neuritis." *J Tradit Chin Med.* 2006; 26: 8–12.

51. Abuaisha, B.B.; Costanzi, J.B.; Boulton, A.J. "Acupuncture for the treatment of chronic painful peripheral diabetic neuropathy: a long-term study." *Diabetes Res Clin Pract.* 1998; 39: 115–121.

52. Wang, Y.P.; Ji, L.; Li, J.T.; et al. "Effects of acupuncture on diabetic peripheral neuropathies." *Zhongguo Zhen Jiu.* 2005; 25: 542–544.

53. Ahn, A.C.; Bennani, T.; Freeman, R.; Hamdy, O.; Kaptchuk, T.J. "Two styles of acupuncture for treating painful diabetic neuropathy—a pilot randomized control trial." *Acupuncture in Medicine.* 2007; 25(1–2): 11–17.

54. Mayer-Davis, E.J.; D'Agostino, R. Jr.; Karter, A.J.,; Haffner, S.M.; Rewers, M.J.; Saad, M.; et al. "Intensity and amount of physical activity in relation to insulin sensitivity: the Insulin Resistance Atherosclerosis Study." *JAMA.* 1998; 279: 669- -674.

55. Lemaster, J.W.; Mueller, M.J.; Reiber, G.E.; Mehr, D.R; Madsen, R.W.; Conn, V.S. "Effect of weight-bearing activity on foot ulcer incidence in peo-

ple with diabetic peripheral neuropathy: feet first randomized controlled trial." *Phys Ther.* 2008; 88(11): 1,385–1,398.

56. Lemaster, J.W.; Mueller, M.J.; Reiber, G.E.; Mehr, D.R.; Madsen, R.W.; Conn, V.S. "Effect of weight-bearing activity on foot ulcer incidence in people with diabetic peripheral neuropathy: feet first randomized controlled trial." *Phys Ther.* 2008; 88(11): 1,385–1,398.

57. Freeman, J.S. "Treating Hispanic patients for type 2 diabetes mellitus: special considerations." *J Am Osteopath Assoc.* 2008; 108(5 Suppl 3): 5–13.

58. Mayer-Davis, E.J.; D'Agostino, R. Jr.; Karter, A.J.; Haffner, S.M.; Rewers, M.J.; Saad, M.; et al. "Intensity and amount of physical activity in relation to insulin sensitivity: the Insulin Resistance Atherosclerosis Study." *JAMA.* 1998; 279: 669–674.

59. Praet, S.F.; Jonkers, R.A.; Schep, G.; Stehouwer, C.D.; Kuipers, H.; Keizer, H.A.; van Loon, L.J. "Long-standing, insulin-treated type 2 diabetes patients with complications respond well to short-term resistance and interval exercise training." *Eur J Endocrinol.* 2008; 158(2): 163–172.

60. Burnfield, J.M.; Jorde, A.G.; Augustin, T.R.; Augustin, T.A.; Bashford, G.R. "Variations in plantar pressure variables across five cardiovascular exercises." *Med Sci Sports Exerc.* 2007; 39(11): 2,012–2,020.

61. Weintraub, M.I.; Cole, S.P. "Pulsed magnetic field therapy in refractory neuropathic pain secondary to peripheral neuropathy: electrodiagnostic parameters—pilot study." *Neurorehabil Neural Repair.* 2004; 18: 42–46.

62. Weintraub, M.I.; Wolfe, G.I.; Barohn, R.A.; et al. "Static magnetic field therapy for symptomatic diabetic neuropathy: a randomized, double-blind, placebo-controlled trial." *Arch Phys Med Rehabil.* 2003; 84: 736–746.

63. Zhao, J.L.; Li, Z.R. "Clinical observation on mild-warm moxibustion for treatment of diabetic peripheral neuropathy." *Zhongguo Zhen Jiu.* 2008; 28(1): 13–16.

64. Malhotra, V.; Singh, S.; Tandon, O.P.; et al. "Effect of Yoga asanas on nerve conduction in type 2 diabetes." *Indian J Physiol Pharmacol.* 2002; 46: 298–306.

65. Yiu, G.; Zhigang, H. "Glial inhibition of CNS axon regeneration." *Nature Reviews Neuroscience.* 2006; 7: 617–627.

Chapter 6

1. American Diabetes Association. "Diabetes: Heart Disease and Stroke." Retrieved October 4, 2008. www.diabetes.org/diabetes-heart-disease-stroke.jsp.

2. Walker, C.; Reamy, B.V. "Diets for cardiovascular disease prevention: what is the evidence?" *Am Fam Physician*. 2009; 79(7): 571–578.

3. Mente, A.; de Koning, L.; Shannon, H.S.; Anand, S.S. "A systematic review of the evidence supporting a causal link between dietary factors and coronary heart disease." *Arch Intern Med*. 2009; 169(7): 659–669.

4. Mente, A.; de Koning, L.; Shannon, H.S.; Anand, S.S. "A systematic review of the evidence supporting a causal link between dietary factors and coronary heart disease." *Arch Intern Med*. 2009; 169(7): 659–669.

5. Hu, F.B.; Rimm, E.B.; Stampfer, M.J.; Ascherio, A.; Spiegelman, D.; Willett, W.C. "Prospective study of major dietary patterns and risk of coronary heart disease in men." *Am J Clin Nutr*. 2000; 72(4): 912–921.

6. Liu, S.; Manson, J.E.; Lee, I.M.; Cole, S.R.; Hennekens, C.H.; Willett, W.C.; Buring, J.E. "Fruit and vegetable intake and risk of cardiovascular disease: the Women's Health Study." *Am J Clin Nutr*. 2000; 72(4): 922–928.

7. Mente, A.; de Koning, L.; Shannon, H.S.; Anand, S.S. "A systematic review of the evidence supporting a causal link between dietary factors and coronary heart disease." *Arch Intern Med*. 2009; 169(7): 659–669.

8. American Heart Association. "Diet & Nutrition." www.american-heart.org/presenter.jhtml?identifier=1200010.

9. Walker, C.; Reamy, B.V. "Diets for cardiovascular disease prevention: what is the evidence?" *Am Fam Physician*. 2009; 79(7): 571–578.

10. Englisch, W.; Beckers, C.; Unkauf, M.; et al. "Efficacy of Artichoke dry extract in patients with hyperlipoproteinemia." *Arzneimittelforschung*. 2000; 50: 260–265.

11. Pittler, M.H.; Thompson, C.O.; Ernst, E. "Artichoke leaf extract for treating hypercholesterolaemia." *Cochrane Database Syst Rev*. 2002; 3: CD003335.

12. Becker, M.; Staab, D.; Von Bergmann, K. "Treatment of severe familial hypercholesterolemia in childhood with sitosterol and sitostanol." *J Pediatr*. 1993; 122: 292–296.

13. Oster, P.; Schlierf, G.; Heuck, C.C.; et al. "Sitosterol in familial hyperlipoproteinemia type II. A randomized, double-blind, cross-over study." *Dtsch Med Wochenschr*. 1976; 101: 1.308–1.311.

14. Schlierf, G.; Oster, P.; Heuck, C.C.; et al. "Sitosterol in juvenile type II hyperlipoproteinemia." *Atherosclerosis*. 1978; 30: 245–248.

15. Schwartzkopff, W.; Jantke, H.J. "Dose-effect of beta-sitosterin in type IIa and IIb hypercholesterolemias." *MMW Munch Med Wochenschr*. 1978; 120: 1,575–1,578.

16. Becker, M.; Staab, D.; Von Bergman, K. "Long-term treatment of severe

familial hypercholesterolemia in children: effect of sitosterol and bezafibrate." *Pediatrics*. 1992; 89: 138–142.

17. Weststrate, J.A.; Meijer, G.W. "Plant sterol-enriched margarines and reduction of plasma total- and LDL-cholesterol concentrations in normocholesterolaemic and mildly hypercholesterolaemic subjects." *Eur J Clin Nutr*. 1998; 52: 334–343.

18. Anon. "FDA authorizes new coronary heart disease health claim for plant sterol and plant stanol esters." FDA, 2000.

19. Lichtenstein, A.H.; Deckelbaum, R.J. "Stanol/sterol ester-containing foods and blood cholesterol levels: a statement for healthcare professionals." Nutrition Committee, Council on Nutrition, Physical Activity, Metabolism of American Heart Association. *Circulation*. 2001; 103: 1,177–1,179.

20. Matvienko, O.A.; Lewis, D.S.; Swanson, M.; et al. "A single daily dose of soybean phytosterols in ground beef decreases serum total cholesterol and LDL cholesterol in young, mildly hypercholesterolemic men." *Am J Clin Nutr*. 2002; 76: 57–64.

21. Neil, H.A.; Meijer, G.W.; Roe, L.S. "Randomised controlled trial of use by hypercholesterolaemic patients of a vegetable oil sterol-enriched fat spread." *Atherosclerosis*. 2001; 156: 329–337.

22. Pepping, J. "Coenzyme Q10." *Am J Health-Syst Pharm*. 1999; 56: 519–521.

23. Hodgson, J.M.; Watts, G.F.; Playford, D.A.; et al. "Coenzyme Q10 improves blood pressure and glycaemic control: a controlled trial in subjects with type 2 diabetes." *Eur J Clin Nutr*. 2002; 56: 1,137–1,142.

24. Singh, R.B.; Niaz, M.A.; Rastogi, S.S.; et al. "Effect of hydrosoluble coenzyme Q10 on blood pressures and insulin resistance in hypertensive patients with coronary artery disease." *J Hum Hypertens*. 1999; 13: 203–208.

25. Langsjoen, P.; Willis, R.; Folkers, K. "Treatment of essential hypertension with coenzyme Q10." *Mol Aspects Med*. 1994; 265–272.

26. Hsu, C.H.; Tsai, T.H.; Kao, Y.H.; Hwang, K.C.; Tseng, T.Y.; Chou, P. "Effect of green tea extract on obese women: a randomized, double-blind, placebo-controlled clinical trial." *Clin Nutr*. 2008; 27(3): 363–370.

27. Nagao, T.; Hase, T.; Tokimitsu, I. "A green tea ext ract high in catechins reduces body fat and cardiovascular risks in humans." *Obesity*. 2007; 15(6): 1,473–1,483.

28. Maron, D.J.; Lu, G.P.; Cai, N.S.; et al. "Cholesterol-lowering effect of a theaflavin-enriched green tea extract: a randomized controlled trial." *Arch Intern Med*. 2003; 163: 1,448–1,453

29. Iso, H.; Date, C.; Wakai, K.; et al. JACC Study Group. "The relationship

between green tea and total caffeine intake and risk for self-reported type 2 diabetes among Japanese adults." *Ann Intern Med.* 2006; 144: 554–562.

30. Gaddi, A.; Descovich, G.C.; Noseda, G.; et al. "Controlled evaluation of pantethine, a natural hypolipidemic compound, in patients with different forms of hyperlipoproteinemia." *Atherosclerosis.* 1984; 50: 73–83.

31. Gaddi, A.; Descovich, G.C.; Noseda, G.; et al. "Controlled evaluation of pantethine, a natural hypolipidemic compound, in patients with different forms of hyperlipoproteinemia." *Atherosclerosis.* 1984; 50: 73–83.

32. Angelico, M.; Pinto, G.; Ciaccheri, C.; et al. "Improvement in serum lipid profile in hyperlipoproteinaemic patients after treatment with pantethine: a crossover, double-blind trial versus placebo." *Curr Ther Res.* 1983; 33: 1,091–1,097.

33. Bertolini, S.; Donati, C.; Elicio, N.; et al. "Lipoprotein changes induced by pantethine in hyperlipoproteinemic patients: adults and children." *Int J Clin Pharmacol Ther Toxicol.* 1986; 24: 630–637.

34. Arsenio, L.; Caronna, S.; Lateana, M.; et al. "Hyperlipidemia, diabetes and atherosclerosis: Efficacy of treatment with pantethine." *Acta Biomed Ateneo Parmense.* 1984; 55: 25–42.

35. Donati, C.; Barbi, G.; Cairo, G.; et al. "Pantethine improves the lipid abnormalities of chronic hemodialysis patients: Results of a multicenter clinical trial." *Clin Nephrol.* 1986; 25: 70–74.

36. Donati, C.; Bertieri, R.S.; Barbi, G. "Pantethine, diabetes mellitus and atherosclerosis. Clinical study of 1045 patients." *Clin Ter.* 1989; 128: 411–422.

37. Coronel, G.; Tornero, F.; Torrente, J.; et al. "Treatment of hyperlipidemia in diabetic patients on dialysis with a physiological substance." *Am J Nephrol.* 1991; 11: 32–36.

38. Nguyen, T.T.; Dale, L.C.; von Bergmann, K.; Croghan, I.T. "Cholesterol-lowering effect of stanol ester in a US population of mildly hypercholesterolemic men and women: a randomized controlled trial." *Mayo Clin Proc.* 1999; 74: 1,198–1,206.

39. Vuorio, A.F.; Gylling, H.; Turtola, H.; et al. "Stanol ester margarine alone and with simvastatin lowers serum cholesterol in families with familial hypercholesterolemia caused by the FH-north karelia mutation." *Arterioscler Thromb Vasc Biol.* 2000; 20: 500–506.

40. Weststrate, J.A.; Meijer, G.W. "Plant sterol-enriched margarines and reduction of plasma total- and LDL-cholesterol concentrations in normocholesterolaemic and mildly hypercholesterolaemic subjects." *Eur J Clin Nutr.* 1998; 52: 334–343.

41. Gylling, H.; Miettinen, T.A. "Cholesterol reduction by different plant stanol mixtures and with variable fat intake." *Metabolism.* 1999; 48: 575–580.

42. Gylling, H.; Puska, P.; Vartiainen, E.; et al. "Serum sterols during stanol ester feeding in a mildly hypercholesterolemic population." *J Lipid Res.* 1999; 40: 593–600.

43. Gylling, H.; Radhakrishnan, R.; Miettinen, T.A. "Reduction of serum cholesterol in postmenopausal women with previous myocardial infarction and cholesterol malabsorption induced by dietary sitostanol ester margarine: women and dietary sitostanol." *Circulation.* 1997; 96: 4,226–4,231.

44. Gylling, H.; Miettinen, T.A. "Serum cholesterol and cholesterol and lipoprotein metabolism in hypercholesterolaemic NIDDM patients before and during sitostanol ester-margarine treatment." *Diabetologia.* 1994; 37: 773–780.

45. Gylling, H.; Miettinen, T.A. "Effects of inhibiting cholesterol absorption and synthesis on cholesterol and lipoprotein metabolism in hypercholesterolemic non-insulin-dependent diabetic men." *J Lipid Res.* 1996; 37: 1,776–1,785.

46. Gylling, H.; Puska, P.; Vartiainen, E.; et al. "Retinol, vitamin D, carotenes and alpha-tocopherol in serum of a moderately hypercholesterolemic population consuming sitostanol ester margarine." *Am J Cardiol.* 1999; 145: 279–285.

47. Hallikainen, M.A.; Uusitupa, M.I. "Effects of 2 low-fat stanol ester-containing margarines on serum cholesterol concentrations as part of a low-fat diet in hypercholesterolemic subjects." *Am J Clin Nutr.* 1999; 69: 403–410.

48. Jones, P.J.; Ntanios, F.Y.; Raeini-Sarjaz, M.; et al. "Cholesterol-lowering efficacy of a sitostanol-containing phytosterol mixture with a prudent diet in hyperlipidemic men." *Am J Clin Nutr.* 1999; 69: 1,144–1,150.

49. Gylling, H.; Siimes, M.A.; Miettinen, T.A. "Sitostanol ester margarine in dietary treatment of children with familial hypercholesterolemia." *J Lipid Res.* 1995; 36: 1,807–1,812.

50. Miettinen, T.A.; Puska, P.; Gylling, H.; et al. "Reduction of serum cholesterol with sitostanol-ester margarine in a mildly hypercholesterolemic population." *N Engl J Med.* 1995; 333(20): 1,308–1,312.

51. Vanhanen, H.T.; Kajander, J.; Lehtovirta, H. "Serum levels, absorption efficiency, faecal elimination and synthesis of cholesterol during increasing doses of dietary sitostanol esters in hypercholesterolaemic subjects." *Clin Sci.* 1994; 87: 61–67.

52. Plat, J.; van Onselen, E.N.; van Heugten, M.M.; Mensink, R.P. "Effects

on serum lipids, lipoproteins and fat soluble antioxidant concentrations of consumption frequency of margarines and shortenings enriched with plant stanol esters." *Eur J Clin Nutr.* 2000; 54: 671–677.

53. Hallikainen, M.A.; Sarkkinen, E.S.; Gylling, H.; et al. "Comparison of the effects of plant sterol ester and plant stanol ester-enriched margarines in lowering serum cholesterol concentrations in hypercholesterolaemic subjects on a low-fat diet." *Eur J Clin Nutr.* 2000; 54: 715–725.

54. Law, M. "Plant sterol and stanol margarines and health." *BMJ.* 2000; 320: 861–864.

55. Lichtenstein, A.H.; Deckelbaum, R.J. "Stanol/sterol ester-containing foods and blood cholesterol levels: a statement for healthcare professionals from Nutrition Committee, Council on Nutrition, Physical Activity, Metabolism of American Heart Association." *Circulation.* 2001; 103: 1,177–1,779.

56. Chu, Q.; Wang, L.; Liu, G.Z. "Clinical observation on acupuncture for treatment of diabetic nephropathy." *Zhongguo Zhen Jiu.* 2007; 27(7):488–490.

57. Liao, H.; Xi, P.; Chen Q.; Yi, L.; Zhao, Y. "Clinical study on acupuncture, moxibustion, acupuncture plus moxibustion at Weiwanxiashu (EX-B3) for treatment of diabetes." *Zhongguo Zhen Jiu.* 2007; 27(7): 482–484.

58. Cabio_lu, M.T.; Ergene, N. "Electroacupuncture therapy for weight loss reduces serum total cholesterol, triglycerides, and LDL cholesterol levels in obese women." *Am J Chin Med.* 2005; 33(4): 525–533.

59. Sample Adult Core component of the 1997-2001 National Health Interview Surveys. Figure 7.1. "Percent of adults aged 18 years and over who engaged in regular leisure-time physical activity: United States, 1997-2001." *CDC National Center for Health Statistics.*

60. American Heart Association. "Exercise and Fitness." July 21, 2008. Retrieved May 15, 2009. www.americanheart.org/presenter.jhtml?identifier=1200013.

61. Kokkinos, P.F.; Giannelou, A.; Manolis, A.; Pittaras, A. "Physical activity in the prevention and management of high blood pressure." *Hellenic J Cardiol.* 2009; 50(1): 52–59.

62. Lavie, C.J.; Thomas, R.J.; Squires, R.W.; Allison, T.G.; Milani, R.V. "Exercise training and cardiac rehabilitation in primary and secondary prevention of coronary heart disease." *Mayo Clin Proc.* 2009; 84 (4): 373–383.

63. Lee, I.M., et al. "Exercise and Risk of Stroke in Male Physicians." *Stroke.* 1999; 30: 1–6.

64. Cardenas, G.A.; Lavie, C.J.; Cardenas, V.; Milani, R.V.; McCullough,

P.A. "The importance of recognizing and treating low levels of high-density lipoprotein cholesterol: a new era in atherosclerosis management." *Rev Cardiovasc Med.* 2008; 9(4): 239–258.

65. The Transcendental Meditation Program. "The Technique." www.tm.org/meditation-techniques.

66. Rainforthm, M.V.; Schneider, R.H.; Nidich, S.I.; Gaylord-King, C.; Salerno, J.W.; Anderson, J.W. "Stress reduction programs in patients with elevated blood pressure: a systematic review and meta-analysis." *Curr Hypertens Rep.* 2007; 9(6): 520–528.

67. Walton, K.G.; Schneider, R.H.; Nidich, S.I.; Salerno, J.W.; Nordstrom, C.K.; Bairey Merz, C.N. "Psychosocial stress and cardiovascular disease Part 2: effectiveness of the Transcendental Meditation program in treatment and prevention." *Behav Med.* 2002; 28(3): 106–123.

68. Ospina, M.B.; Bond, K.; Karkhaneh, M.; Tjosvold, L.; Vandermeer, B.; Liang, Y.; Bialy, L.; Hooton, N.; Buscemi, N.; Dryden, D.M.; Klassen, T.P. "Meditation practices for health: state of the research." *Evid Rep Technol Assess.* 2007; (155): 1–263.

69. Jain, S.; Agrawal, R.P.; Gahlot, S.; Khatri ,D., Mathur, K.C.. "Effects of yoga and meditation on clinical and biochemical parameters of metabolic syndrome." *Explore.* 2009; 5(3): 147.

70. Bijlani, R.L.; Vempati, R.P.; Yadav, R.K.; Ray, R.B.; Gupta, V.; Sharma, R.; Mehta, N.; Mahapatra, S.C. "A brief but comprehensive lifestyle education program based on yoga reduces risk factors for cardiovascular disease and diabetes mellitus." *J Altern Complement Med.* 2005; 11(2): 267–274.

71. American Diabetes Association. "Stroke." Retrieved October 4, 2008. www.diabetes.org/diabetes-heart-disease-stroke.jsp.

Chapter 7

1. Scovell, S. "Best Treatment for Peripheral Vascular Disease Is Prevention." *DOC News.* 2007; 4(6): 4.

2. Jude, E.B. "Intermittent Claudication in the Patient With Diabetes." *Br J Diabetes Vasc Dis.* 2004; 4(4) :238–242.

3. Jude, E.B. "Intermittent Claudication in the Patient With Diabetes." *Br J Diabetes Vasc Dis.* 2004; 4(4): 238–242.

4. Kiesewetter, H.; Jung, F.; Jung, E.M.; et al. "Effects of garlic coated tablets in peripheral arterial occlusive disease." *Clin Investig.* 1993; 71: 383–386.

5. Pittler, M.H.; Ernst, E. "Ginkgo biloba extract for the treatment of intermittent claudication: a meta-analysis of randomized trials." *Am J Med.* 2000; 108: 276–281.

6. Schweizer, J.; Hautmann, C. "Comparison of two dosages of Ginkgo biloba extract Egb 761 in patients with peripheral arterial occlusive disease Fontain's stage llb / a randomised, double-blind, multicentric clinical trial." *Arzneimittelforschung*. 1999; 49: 900–904.

7. Li, A.L.; Shi, Y.D.; Landsmann, B.; et al. "Hemorheology and walking of peripheral arterial occlusive diseases patients during treatment with Gingko biloba extract." *Chung Kuo Yao Li Hsueh Pao*. 1998; 19: 417–421.

8. Sunderland, G.T.; Belch, J.J.; Sturrock, R.D.; et al. "A double-blind, randomized, placebo-controlled trial of hexopal in primary Raynaud's disease." *Clin Rheumatol*. 1988; 7: 46–49.

9. Holti, G. "An experimentally controlled evaluation of the effect of inositol nicotinate upon the digital blood flow in patients with Raynaud's phenomenon." *J Int Med Res*. 1979; 7: 473–483.

10. Ring, E.F.; Bacon, P.A. "Quantitative thermographic assessment of inositol nicotinate therapy in Raynaud's phenomena." *J Int Med Res*. 1977; 5: 217–222.

11. Brevetti, G.; Chiariello, M.; Ferulano, G.; et al. "Increases in walking distance in patients with peripheral vascular disease treated with L-carnitine: a double-blind, cross-over study." *Circulation*. 1988; 77: 767–773.

12. Brevetti, G.; Diehm, C.; Lambert, D.; et al. "European multicenter study on propionyl-L-carnitine in intermittent claudication." *J Am Coll Cardiol*. 1999; 34: 1,618–1,624.

13. Brevetti, G.; Pe rna, S.; Sabba, C.; et al. "Propionyl-L-carnitine in intermittent claudication: double-blind, placebo-controlled, dose titration, multicenter study." *J Am Coll Cardiol*. 1995; 26: 1,411–1,416.

14. Brevetti, G.; Perna, S.; Sabba, C.; et al. "Effect of propionyl-L-carnitine on quality of life in intermittent claudication." *Am J Cardiol*. 1997; 79: 777–780.

15. Brevetti, G.; Perna, S.; Sabba, C.; et al. "Superiority of L-propionylcarnitine vs L-carnitine in improving walking capacity in patients with peripheral vascular disease: an acute, intravenous, double-blind, cross-over study." *Eur Heart J*. 1992; 13: 251–255.

16. Dal Lago, A.; De Martini, D.; Flore, R.; et al. "Effects of propionyl-L-carnitine on peripheral arterial obliterative disease of the lower limbs: a double-blind clinical trial." *Drugs Exp Clin Res*. 1999; 25: 29–36.

17. Hiatt, W.R.; Regensteiner, J.G.; Creager, M.A.; et al. "Propionyl-L-carnitine improves exercise performance and functional status in patients with claudication." *Am J Med*. 2001; 110: 616–622.

18. Dal Lago, A.; De Martini, D.; Flore, R.; et al. "Effects of propionyl-L-carnitine on peripheral arterial obliterative disease of the lower limbs: a double-blind clinical trial." *Drugs Exp Clin Res.* 1999; 25: 29–36.

19. Castano, G.; Mas, R.; Roca, J.; et al. "A double-blind, placebo-controlled study of the effects of policosanol in patients with intermittent claudication." *Angiology.* 1999; 50: 123–130.

20. Castano, G.; Mas Ferreiro, R.; Fernandez, L.; et al. "A long-term study of policosanol in the treatment of intermittent claudication." *Angiology.* 2001; 52: 115–125.

21. Carbajal, D.; Arruzazabala, M.L.; Valdes, S.; Mas Ferreiro, R. "Effect of policosanol on platelet aggregation and serum levels of arachidonic acid metabolites in healthy volunteers." *Prostaglandins Leukot Essent Fatty Acids.* 1998; 58: 61–64.

22. Arruzazabala, M.L.; Valdes, S.; Mas, R.; et al. "Effect of policosanol successive dose increases on platelet aggregation in healthy volunteers." *Pharmacol Res.* 1996; 34: 181–185.

23. Haeger, K. "Long-time treatment of intermittent claudication with vitamin E." *Am J Clin Nutr.* 1974; 27: 1,179–1,181.

24. Williams, H.T.; Fenna, D.; Macbeth, R.A. "Alpha tocopherol in the treatment of intermittent claudication." *Surg Gynecol Obstet.* 1971; 662–666.

25. Piesse, J.W. "Vitamin E and peripheral vascular disease." *Int Clin Nutr Rev.* 1984; 4: 178–182.

26. Pittler, M.H.; Ernst, E. "Complementary therapies for peripheral arterial disease: systematic review." *Atherosclerosis.* 2005; 181(1): 1–7.

27. Li, X.; Hirokawa, M.; Inoue, Y.; Sugano, N.; Qian, S.; Iwai, T. "Effects of acupressure on lower limb blood flow for the treatment of peripheral arterial occlusive diseases." *Surg Today.* 2007; 37(2): 103–108.

28. Solun, M.N.; Lia_fer, A.I. "Acupuncture in the treatment of diabetic angiopathy of the lower extremities." *Probl Endokrinol.* 1991; 37(4): 20–23.

29. Rice, B.; Kalker, A.J.; Schindler, J.V.; Dixon, R.M. "Effect of Biofeedback-Assisted Relaxation Training on Foot Ulcer Healing." *J Am Podiatr Med Assoc.* 2001; 91: 132–141.

30. Galper, D.I.; Taylor, A.G.; Cox, D.J. "Current status of mind-body interventions for vascular complications of diabetes." *Fam Community Health.* 2003; 26(1): 34–40.

31. Saunders, J.T.; Cox, D.J.; Teates, C.D.; Pohl, S.L. "Thermal biofeedback in the treatment of intermittent claudication in diabetes: a case study." *Biofeedback Self Regul.* 1994; 19(4): 337–345.

32. Shamoun, F.; Sural, N.; Abela, G. "Peripheral artery disease: therapeutic advances." *Expert Rev Cardiovasc Ther.* 2008; 6(4): 539–553.

33. Watson, L.; Ellis, B.; Leng, G.C. "Exercise for intermittent claudication." *Cochrane Database Syst Rev.* 2008; (4): CD000990.

34. Seals, D.R.; Desouza, C.A.; Donato, A.J.; Tanaka, H. "Habitual exercise and arterial aging." *J Appl Physiol.* 2008; 105(4): 1,323–1,332.

Chapter 8

1. Pardianto, G. et al. "Understanding diabetic retinopathy." *Mimbar Ilmiah Oftalmologi.* Indonesia. 2005; 2: 65–66.

2. American Diabetes Association. "Diabetic Retinopathy." Viewed October 25, 2008. http://professional.diabetes.org/Disease_Backgrounder. aspx?TYP=6&MID=300.

3. Brazionis, L.; Rowley, Sr. K.; Itsiopoulos, C.; Harper, C.A.; O'Dea, K. "Homocysteine and Diabetic Retinopathy." *Diabetes Care.* 2008; 31: 50–56.

4. Anonymous. "Vacci nium myrtillus (bilberry) monograph." *Altern Med Rev.* 2001; 6(5): 500–504.

5. Scharrer, A.; Ober, M. "Anthocyanosides in the treatment of retinopathies." *Klin Monatabl Augenheilkd.* 1981; 178: 386–389.

6. Mian, E.; Curri, S.B.; Lietti, A.; Bombardelli, E. "Anthocyanosides and the walls of the microvessels: further aspects of the mechanism of action of their protective effect in syndromes due to abnormal capillary fragility." *Minerva Med.* 1977; 68: 3,565-3,581.

7. "Vaccinium myrtillus (Bilberry) Monograph." *Alternative Medicine Review.* 2001; 6(5): 500–504.

8. Perossini, M.; Guidi, G.; Chiellini, S.; Siravo, D. "Diabetic and hypertensive retinopathy therapy with Vaccinium myrtillus anthocyanosides (Tegens). Double blind, placebo-controlled clinical trial." *Ann Ottalmol Clin Ocul.* 1987; 113: 1,173–1,177.

9. Scharrer, A.; Ober, M. "Anthocyanosides in the treatment of retinopathies." *Kiln Monastbl Augenheilkd.* 1981; 178: 386–389.

10. Lanthony, P.; Cosson JP. "The course of color vision in early diabetic retinopathy treated with ginkgo biloba extract." A preliminary, double-blind versus placebo study. *J Fr Ophtalmol.* 1988; 11: 671–674.

11. Huang, S.Y.; Jeng, C.; Kao, S.C.; Yu, J.J.; Liu, D.Z. "Improved haemorrheological properties by Ginkgo biloba extract (Egb 761) in type 2 diabetes mellitus complicated with retinopathy." *Clin Nutr.* 2004; 23(4): 615–621.

12. Spadea, L.; Balestrazzi, E. "Treatment of vascular retinopathies with pycnogenol." *Phytother Res.* 2001; 15: 219–223.

13. "Oligomeric Proanthocyanidins (OPCs) Monograph." *Alternative Medicine Review.* 2003; 8(4): 442–450.

14. Froantin, M. "Procyanidolic oligomers in the treatment of capillary fragility and retinopathy in diabetics." *Med Int.* 1981; 16: 432–434.

15. Mohammed Ismail, S.A.; Fahmy, I.A.; Farrag, S.A.M. "Inverse Correlation of Low Vitamin B_{12}, Folic Acid and Homocysteine Levels in Diabetic Retinopathy." *Turk J Biochem.* 2008; 33(1): 14–18.

16. Kornerup, T.; Strom, L. "Vitamin B_{12} and retinopathy in juvenile diabetics." *Acta Paediatr.* 1958; 47: 646–651.

17. Brazionis, L.; Rowley Sr., K.; Itsiopoulos, C., Harper, C.A.; O'Dea, K. "Homocysteine and Diabetic Retinopathy." *Diabetes Care.* 2008; 31: 50–56.

18. Homocysteine Lowering Trialists' Collaboration. "Lowering blood homocysteine with folic acid based supplements: meta-analysis of randomized trials." *BMJ.* 1998; 316: 894–898.

19. Zhang, Z.L.; Ji, X.Q.; Zhang, Y.H.; Yu, S.H.; Xue, L. "Controlled study on the needling method for regulating the spleen and stomach for treatment of diabetic retinopathy." *Zhongguo Zhen Jiu.* 2006; 26(12): 839–842.

20. Lu, J.G.; Friberg, T.R. "Idiopathic central serous retinopathy in China: a report of 600 cases (624 eyes) treated by acupuncture." *Ophthalmic Surg.* 1987; 18(8): 608–611.

21. Zhu, X.; Bi, A.; Han, X. "Treatment of retinal vein obstruction with acupuncture and Chinese medicinal herbs." *J Tradit Chin Med.* 2002; 22(3): 211–213.

22. Chen, Y. "Magnets on ears helped diabetics." *Am J Chin Med.* 2002; 30(1): 183–185.

23. Siero_, A.; Cie_lar, G. "Application of variable magnetic fields in medicine." *Wiad Lek.* 2003; 56(9–10): 434–441.

Chapter 9

1. American Diabetes Association. "Obesity." Retrieved October 23, 2008. http://professional.diabetes.org/Disease_Backgrounder.aspx?TYP=6&MID=267.

2. American Diabetes Association. "Goals of Treatment." http://professional.diabetes.org/Disease_Backgrounder.aspx?MID=309&RD=1.

3. Saperstein, S.L.; Atkinson, N.L.; Gold, R.S. "The impact of Internet use for weight loss." *Obes Rev.* 2007; 8(5): 459–465.

4. Weinstein, P.K. "A review of weight loss programs delivered via the Internet." *J Cardiovasc Nurs.* 2006; 21(4): 251–258.

5. Körtke, H.; Frisch, S.; Zittermann, A.; et al. "A telemetrically-guided program for weight reduction in overweight subjects (the SMART study)." *Dtsch Med Wochenschr.* 2008; 133(24): 1,297–1,303.

6. Frisard, M.I.; Greenway, F.L.; Delany, J.P. "Comparison of methods to assess body composition changes during a period of weight loss." *Obes Res.* 2005; 13(5): 845–854.

7. Bowerman, S.; Bellman, M.; Saltsman, P.; et al. "Implementation of a primary care physician network obesity management program." *Obes Res.* 2001; 9Suppl4: 321S—325S.

8. Weiner, S. "The addiction of overeating: self-help groups as treatment models." *J Clin Psychol.* 1998; 54(2): 163–167.

9. Wasson, D.H.; Jackson, M. "An analysis of the role of overeaters anonymous in women's recovery from bulimia nervosa." *Eat Disord.* 2004; 12(4): 337–356.

10. Rorty, M.; Yager, J.; Rossotto, E. "Why and how do women recover from bulimia nervosa? The subjective appraisals of forty women recovered for a year or more." *Int J Eat Disord.* 1993; 14(3): 249–260.

11. Miller-Kovach, K.; Hermann, M.; Winick, M. "The psychological ramifications of weight management." *J Womens Health Gend Based Med.* 1999; 8(4): 477–482.

12. Lowe, M.R.; Kral, T.V.; Miller-Kovach, K. "Weight-loss maintenance 1, 2 and 5 years after successful completion of a weight-loss programme." *Br J Nutr.* 2008; 99(4): 925–930.

13. Kuriyan, R.; Raj, T.; Srinivas, S.K.; Vaz, M.; Rajendran, R.; Kurpad, A.V. "Effect of Caralluma fimbriata extract on appetite, food intake and anthropometry in adult Indian men and women." *Appetite.* 2007; 48(3): 338–344.

14. Kuriyan, R.; Raj, T.; Srinivas, S.K.; Vaz, M.; Rajendran, R.; Kurpad, A.V. "Effect of Caralluma fimbriata extract on appetite, food intake and anthropometry in adult Indian men and women." *Appetite.* 2007; 48(3): 338–344.

15. Lawrence, R.M.; Choudhary, S. "Caralluma fimbriata in the treatment of obesity." Western Geriatric Research Institute, Los Angeles, California.

16. Preuss, H. "Slimaluma(tm): A New Appetite Suppressant Ingredient." Gencor Pacific; 2004.

17. Oben, J.E.; Ngondi, J.L.; Momo, C.N.; Agbor, G.A.; Sobgui, C.S.M. "The use of a Cissus quadrangularis/Irvingia gabonensis combination in the

management of weight loss: a double-blind placebo-controlled study." *Lipids in health and disease.* 2008; 7: 12.

18. Oben, J.; Enyegue, D.M.; Fomekong, G.; et al. "The effect of Cissus quadrangularis (CQR-300) and a Cissus formulation (CORE) on obesity and obesity-induced oxidative stress." *Lipids Health Dis.* 2007; 6: 4.

19. Oben, J.; Kuate, D.; Agbor, G.; et al. "The use of a Cissus quadrangularis formulation in the management of weight loss and metabolic syndrome." *Lipids Health Dis.* 2006; 5: 24.

20. Badmaev, V.; Majeed, M.; Conte, A.A.; Parker, J.E. "Diterpene Forskolin (Coleus forskohlii, Benth.): A possible new compound for reduction of body weight by increasing lean body mass." *Nutra Cos.* 2002; March/April: 6–7.

21. Bhagwat, A.M.; Joshi, B.; Joshi, A.; et al. "A randomized double-blind clinical trial to investigate the efficacy and safety of ForsLean in increasing lean body mass." Mumbai, India: Shri C.B. Patel Research Center for Chemistry and Biological Sciences, 2004.

22. Godard, M.; Johnson, B.; Richmond, S. "Body composition and hormonal adaptations associated with forskolin consumption in overweight and obese men." *Obesity Res.* 2005; 13(8): 1,335–1,343.

23. Tsuguyoshi, A. "Clinical report on root extract of perilla plant (Coleus forskohlii) ForsLean(r) in reducing body fat." Tokyo: Ansano Institute for Sabinsa Corporation, 2001.

24. Henderson, S.; Magu, B.; Rasmussen, C.; et al. "Effects of Coleus Forskohlii Supplementation on Body Composition and Hematological Profiles in Mildly Overweight Women." *Journal of the International Society of Sports Nutrition.* 2005; 2(2): 54–62.

25. Mori, T.A.; Bao, D.Q.; Burke, V.; et al. "Dietary fish as a major component of a weight-loss on serum lipids, Glucose, and insulin metabolism in overweight hypertensive subjects." *Am J Clin Nutr.* 1999; 70: 817–825.

26. Hill, A.M.; Buckley, J.D.; Murphy, K.J.; Howe, P.R. "Combining fish-oil supplements with regular aerobic exercise improves body composition and cardiovascular disease risk factors." *Am J Clin Nutr.* 2007; 85: 1,267–1,274.

27. Thorsdottir, I.; Tomasson, H.; Gunnarsdottir, I.; Gisladottir, E.; Kiely, M.; Parra, M.D.; Bandarra, N.M.; Schaafsma, G.; Martinéz, J.A. :Randomized trial of weight loss diets for young adults varying in fish and fish oil content." *Int J Obesity.* 2007; 31(10): 1,560–1,566.

28. Couet, C.; Delarue, J.; Ritz, P.; Antoine, J.M.; Lamisse, F. "Effect of dietary fish oil on body fat mass and basal fat oxidation in healthy adults." *Int J Obes.* 1997; 21(8): 637–643.

29. Parra, D.; Ramel, A.; Bandarra, N.; Kiely, M.; Martinez, J.A.; Thordottir, I. "A diet rich in long chain omega 3 fatty acids modulates satiety in overweight and obese volunteers during weight loss." *Appetite*, 2008.

30. Dulloo, A.; Duret, C.; Rohrer, D.; et al. "Efficacy of a gren tea extract rich in catechin polyphenols and caffeine in increasing 24-hour energy expenditure and fat oxidation in humand." *Am J Clin Nutr.* 1999; 70: 1,040–1,045.

31. Chantre, P. and Lairon, D. "Recent findings of green tea extract AR25 (Exolise) and its activity for the treatment of obesity." *Phytomedicine.* 2002; 9: 3–8.

32. Westerterp-Plantenga, M.S.; Lejeune, M.P.G.M.; Kovacs, E.M.R. "Body Weight Loss and Weight Maintenance in Relation to Habitual Caffeine Intake and Green Tea Supplementation." *Obesity Research.* 2005; 13(7): 1,195–1,205.

33. Kovacs, E.; Lejeune, M.; Nijs, I.,; Westerterp-Plantenga, M. "Effects of green tea on weight maintenance after body-weight loss." *Br J Nutr.* 2004; 91: 431–437.

34. Zhang, X. "A clinical survey of acupuncture slimming." *J Tradit Chin Med.* 2008; 28(2): 139–147.

35. Cabÿoglu, M.T.; Ergene, N.; Tan, U. "The treatment of obesity by acupuncture." *Int J Neurosci.* 2006; 116(2): 165–175.

36. Lacey, J.M.; Tershakovec, A.M.; Foster, G.D. "Acupuncture for the treatment of obesity: a review of the evidence." *Int J Obes Relat Metab Disord.* 2003; 27(4): 419–427.

37. Bailey, Covert. *The New Fit or Fat.* Mariner Books, 1991.

38. Malomsoki, J. "Effect of oxyhydromassage therapy on some physiological parameters." *Orv Hetil.* 2009; 150(4): 161–164.

39. Dechamps, A.; Gatta, B.; Bourdel-Marchasson, I.; Tabarin, A.; Roger, P. "Pilot study of a 10-week multidisciplinary Tai Chi intervention in sedentary obese women." *Clin J Sport Med.* 2009; 19(1): 49–53.

40. Benavides, S.; Caballero, J. "Ashtanga yoga for children and adolescents for weight management and psychological well being: an uncontrolled open pilot study." *Complement Ther Clin Pract.* 2009; 15(2): 110–114.

41. Madanmohan; Mahadevan, S.K.; Balakrishnan, S.; Gopalakrishnan, M.; Prakash, E.S. "Effect of six weeks yoga training on weight loss following step test, respiratory pressures, handgrip strength and handgrip endurance in young healthy subjects." *Indian J Physiol Pharmacol.* 2008; 52(2): 164–170.

Chapter 10

1. Enstrom, J.E. "Counterpoint—vitamin C and mortality." *Nutr Today.* 1993; 28: 28–32.

2. Lieberman, S.; Bruning, N. "The Real Vitamin & Mineral Book, Second Edition." Garden City Park, New York: Avery Publishing Group, 1997.

3. Anderson, R.A.; Cheng, N.; Bryden, N.A.; et al. "Elevated intakes of supplemental chromium improve glucose and insulin variables in individuals with type 2 diabetes." *Diabetes.* 1997; 46: 1,786–1,791.

4. USDA National Nutrient Database for Standard Reference. Release 21; 2008.

5. Machlin, L.J.; Brin, M. "Bioequivalence of RRR-alpha- tocopheryl acetate and all-rac-alpha-tocopheryl acetate." *Am J Clin Nutr.* 1981; 34(8): 1,633–1,636.

6. New Chapter. www.newchapter.com/page/whole-food.

7. New Chapter. "Every Man." www.newchapter.com/products/every-man.

8. New Chapter. "Every Man." www.newchapter.com/products/every-man.

9. Weis, M.; Mortensen, S.A.; Rassing, M.R.; et al. "Bioavailability of four oral coenzyme Q10 formulations in healthy volunteers." *Mol Aspects Med.* 1994; 15: 273–280.

10. Department of Health and Human Services, Food and Drug Administration. "Facts About Current Good Manufacturing Practices (cGMPs)." Last updated: July 10, 2009. Retrieved July 18, 2009.

11. Department of Health and Human Services, Food and Drug Administration. "Current Good Manufacturing Practice in Manufacturing, Packaging, Labeling, or Holding Operations for Dietary Supplements." 21 CFR Part 111 [Docket No. 1996N–0417] (formerly Docket No. 96N–0417). RIN 0910–AB88; June 2, 2007.

Appendix A

1. "Slow-carb" is a term coined by Patricia and Harvey Haakonson, MD, authors of *Slow Carb for Life.*

2. Ebbeling, C.B.; Leidig, M.M.; Sinclair, K.B.; et al. "Effects of an ad libitum low-Glycemic load diet on cardiovascular disease risk factors in obese young adults." *Am J Clin Nutr.* 2005; 81(5): 976–982.

3. "Similar beneficial results were seen in weight loss with the Mediterranean diet versus a low-fat diet." *N Engl J Med.* 2008; 359: 229–241.

4. DeNoon, D. "Low Carb Out, Slow Carb In? Researchers Say People Lose Weight on a Low-Glycemic-Load Diet." WebMD Medical News, May 11, 2005. Accessed August 4, 2005.

5. Brand-Miller, J. "Optimizing the cardiovascular outcomes of weight loss." *Am J Clin Nutr.* 2005; 81(5): 949–950.

6. Rolfes, S.R.; Pinna, K.; Whitney, E. *Understanding Normal and Clinical Nutrition, 7th Edition.* Belmont, CA: Thomson Wadsworth, 2006.

7. This menu, the subsequent food choices table, and the diet suggestions thereafter are from my good friend and colleague, Jennifer Hofheins, MS, RD, LD.

Appendix C

1. Chuangui, W. "Chinese Family Acupoint Massage." China: Foreign Language Press, 1992.

2. "Whole Medical Systems: An Overview. Backgrounder." Washington, DC: National Center for Complementary and Alternative Medicine, 2004.

3. "Energy Medicine: An Overview. Backgrounder." Washington, DC: National Center for Complementary and Alternative Medicine, 2004.

4. Sample Adult Core component of the 1997-2001 National Health Interview Surveys. Figure 7.1: "Percent of adults aged 18 years and over who engaged in regular leisure-time physical activity: United States, 1997–2001." CDC National Center for Health Statistics.

5. Freeman, L. "Mosby's Complementary & Alternative Medicine: A Research-Based Approach, 2nd. edition." St. Louis, MO: Mosby, 2004.

6. Natural Standard & Faculty of Harvard Medical School. "Magnet Therapy. Aetna InteliHealth Inc." Last updated May 01, 2008. Retrieved January 28, 2009. www.intelihealth.com/IH/ihtIH/WSIHW000/8513/34968/358833.html?d=dmtContent.

7. Park, R.L. *Voodoo Science: The Road from Foolishness to Fraud.* New York, New York: Oxford University Press, 2000: 58–63.

8. Wanjek, C. *Bad Medicine: misconceptions and misuses revealed from distance healing to vitamin O.* Hoboken, New Jersey: John Wiley & Sons., 2003: 1–253.

9. National Science Foundation, Division of Resources Statistics (2006-02). Science and Engineering Indicators, 2006. Arlington, VA. Chapter 7. www.nsf.gov/statistics/seind06/c7/c7s2.htm#c7s2l3.

10. Skalak, T.C.; Morris, C.E. "Chronic static magnetic field exposure alters microvessel enlargement resulting from surgical intervention." *American Journal of Applied Physiology.* 2007; 103(2): 629-636.

11. Gmitrov, J.; Ohkubo, C.; Okano, H. "Effect of 0.25 T static magnetic field on microcirculation in rabbits." *Bioelectromagnetics.* 2002; 23(23): 224–229.

12. Skalak, T.C.; Morris, C.E. "Acute exposure to a moderate strength static magnetic field reduces edema formation in rats." *American Journal of Physiology: Heart and Circulatory Physiology.* 2008; 294(1): H50–H57.

13. Maki, Melissa (2008-01-02). "Biomedical Engineering Study Demonstrates the Healing Value of Magnets. U.Va. Today. January 1, 2002. Retrieved from www.virginia.edu/uvatoday/newsRelease.php?id=3573.

14. Man, D.; Man, B.; Plosker, H. "The influence of a permanent magnetic field therapy on wound healing in suction lipectomy patients: a double-blind study." *Plastic and Reconstructive Surgery.* 1999; 104(7): 2,261–2,266.

15. Mao-liang, C. "Chinese Acupuncture and Moxibustion." Edinburgh: Elsevier Health Sciences, 1993.

16. Malomsoki, J. "Effect of oxyhydromassage therapy on some physiological parameters." *Orv Hetil.* 2009; 150(4): 161–164.

17. Mayo Clinic Staff. "Tai chi: Improved stress reduction, balance, agility for all." Mayo Foundation for Medical Education and Research. November 15, 2007. Retrieved July 12, 2009. www.mayoclinic.com/health/tai-chi/SA00087.

18. Feuerstein, G. "The Shambhala Guide to Yoga." Boston and London: Shambhala Publications, Inc., 1996.

ABOUT THE AUTHOR

Gene Bruno is the Dean of Academics and a professor at the Huntington College of Health Sciences. For over three decades, he has provided professional services—including education, training, clinical nutrition, and research—to nutrition, herbal, and natural product industries, as well as to the public. His articles on nutrition, herbal medicine, nutraceuticals, and integrative health issues have been published in a variety of trade and consumer magazines, as well as peer-reviewed journals and newsletters.

Gene has two undergraduate diplomas in Nutrition from the American Academy of Nutrition and the American Health Science University, a BHS in Nutrition and an MS in Nutrition from the Huntington College of Health Sciences, a graduate diploma in Herbal Medicine from the Australian College of Phytotherapy, and an MHS in Herbal Medicine from the University of New England. He is currently working on his doctorate in Education at Capella University.

INDEX